Through Their Eyes

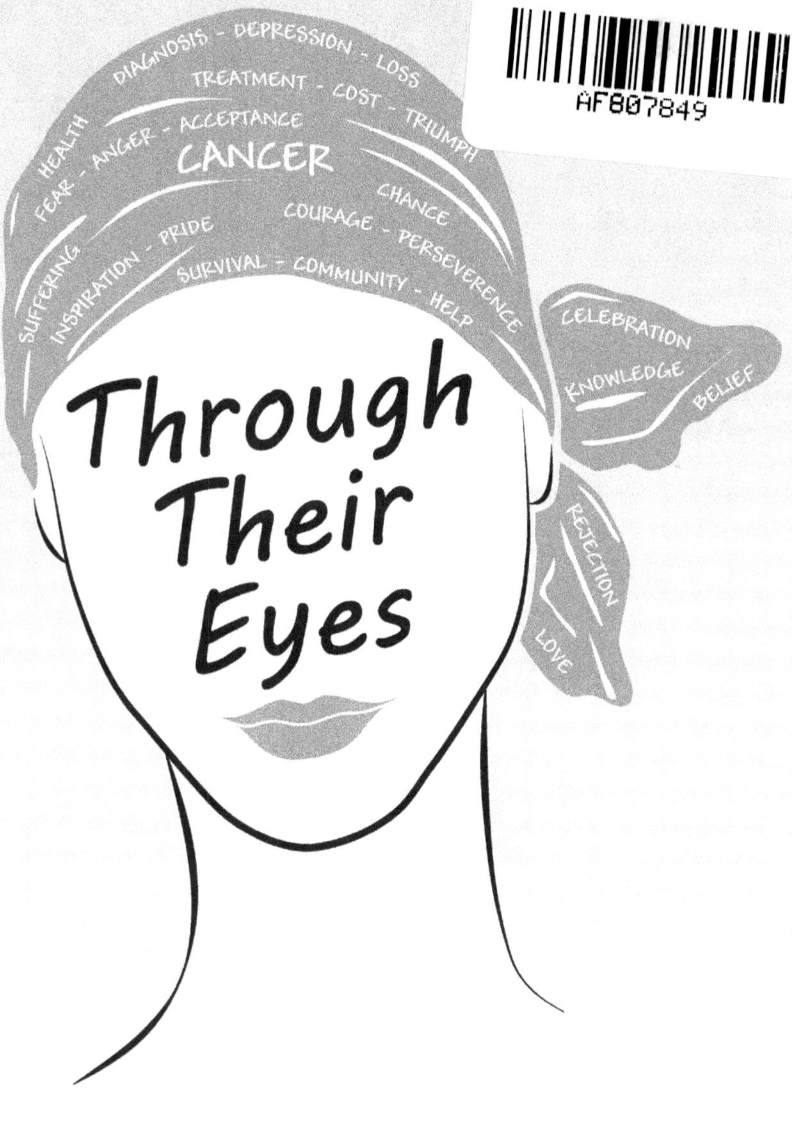

Harshal Mehdi & Aminder Mehdi

outskirtspress
DENVER, COLORADO

Outskirts Press, Inc.
http://www.outskirtspress.com

ISBN: 978-1-4787-5483-1

PRINTED IN THE UNITED STATES OF AMERICA

Introduction

I interviewed nine people for this book. You'll notice that it covers only seven of them. And so, while I have numerous people to thank, I need to start out with an apology: I'm sorry that Helen and Claudia, the first two people I interviewed, are the only people whose stories I never wrote.

I never wrote them because I never had a chance to finish hearing them. Both women had such an inviting, warm way of discussing their lives that I didn't realize how terrifying their disease was for them. In fact, I don't even remember discussing cancer at any length with them. I remember the small things. Like Helen showing off the San Francisco 49ers bandanas she knitted. Or Claudia giggling about her kid's dating life. After I met each of them, I had the same initial thought – *Wow, they look great.* I thought the treatments must have gone really well. I didn't realize initially what an honor and privilege it was to talk with them, and what courage it must have taken for them to openly revisit the course of their disease.

I never got a second meeting with either one. Both died within a month of our introduction. Helen and Claudia taught me to have respect for the disease and the human body. We can withstand a lot and look great, but it can all vanish in such a short time.

When I first found out about their passing, I was upset but also embarrassed. Our discussions had been so nonchalant. Had I trivialized their experiences? Had our conversations actually been too normal?

I hope not. I was afraid to ask them too much about their disease, but in doing so I missed an early opportunity to learn how they managed to discuss their condition with such aplomb.

Society has a penchant for characterizing people by major illness. Of course, if you have the big ailment, you want anything but to be defined by it. This became increasingly evident as I interviewed more people. While everyone was more than willing to talk about their life with cancer, they weren't often willing to let that be the defining aspect of their story. They all felt the other parts of their lives—goals, epiphanies, philosophies—were more central to their being.

Which brings me to the point of this book. No one is ever ready for life-changing events. And medical care can be overwhelmingly complicated for even the most harmless of illnesses. Having a guide would be useful for navigating these unclear waters. So in this book, I hope to do just that, by giving a voice to those that I interviewed. All had been given life-changing diagnoses, and all reacted in ways that are instructive to the rest of us.

What makes a useful guide? For instance, I can't tell you about nausea. I can tell you people get it after chemotherapy, but you probably already know that, if only from how it's perceived en masse through pop culture. And even if I was poetic or eloquent enough to make you feel a person's nausea, how does that help? But if we can delve into the unexpected events, missed opportunities, or even existential crises that accompany a diagnosis, then we have useful experiences to draw upon.

For example, Helen mentioned during our initial conversation how she missed doing household chores like vacuum cleaning or washing the dishes. There was a *rhythm* to life that was suddenly gone. I wrote it down but never placed much importance on it. Some time later, my own grandmother was diagnosed with breast cancer. After chemotherapy, she was fatigued, tired, but never weak enough to stop performing her normal activities. But my family wanted to protect her. "No, don't wash the dishes. Don't cook dinner. Don't do any knitting." Why? We just assumed the less she did, the better off she would be. I've never seen my grandmother in worse shape. Not from a physical point of view, but emotionally she deteriorated. There was nothing left for her to do. And she recovered only when we took the shackles off of her, and let her resume her life. If we had more guidance from experiences like Helen's, then we might have been able to avoid that mess. That is why this book features stories from different people dealing with a cancer diagnosis. I thank everyone who was kind enough to share their experiences so that others might benefit from them.

All this is not to say that the medical aspect of oncology is irrelevant. Whether you want to know it or not, once you're diagnosed, you are required to know the basic elements of this new world. You won't be able to remember every detail your doctor tells you in the office. And relying on the internet can be risky. While there's a lot of good information out there, you never know what you'll get when you google medical therapies. Even the statistics can be very misleading. So with every story I'll teach a little about the basic facts of medical oncology. I repeat some information quite often with the aim of making readers comfortable with medical facts. With every story, the amount of medical description will go down until we're left with only the stories themselves.

I'm just starting out my medical career, so I couldn't have done this on my own. I'd like to thank my friend Michael Dorazio for designing the cover. I thank my family for supporting me, but I am especially grateful for my dad's help. He's been a practicing oncologist for more than twenty years. His name is on the front because without him this wouldn't have been possible—not just for the medical knowledge but also for giving me an up-front look at how much good can be done for people who are truly suffering.

Lastly, to those who have been diagnosed with cancer or who have loved ones with the diagnosis, I wish you the best of luck. I hope this book provides you at least a little help, guidance, and comfort in your journey.

—Harshal Mehdi

Table of Contents

Iron Mike... 1
Marty the Martyr 35
The Snowball 83
It's (Not) Textbook 123
The Other Way 152
The Age-Old Question 184

Iron Mike

VENICE, ITALY'S LEGENDARY island city, is a dream vacation for many. But as Mike and Mary sat in a water taxi off the dock by the airport, they weren't admiring the water canals or the speedboats racing from pier to pier. Their eyes were peeled to their boat's tarmac. It had been raining from the moment they landed and now the blue tarp above them was sagging from the water collecting on it. They watched as the puddle swished from side to side, as the hooks buckled wildly, threatening to give way and drench everyone—and, more importantly, everyone's luggage.

When they were planning the trip, they hadn't even entertained the thought of bad weather. For a brief moment, though, they forgot about the rain and the water balloon above their heads as their taxi pulled up to St. Mark's Plaza, basically the tourist center of the city. Their driver pulled them up to a dock at the plaza. It was absent the numerous hordes of tourists that normally occupy it.

The driver ushered them out. "Your hotel is close to here," he told them. Mike and Mary looked outside, unsure of where to go. As they would soon find out, Venice is a nightmare to navigate. The city's addresses don't follow any logical order. You can go from 15 Paisano Road, cross the alley and you'll end up in 500 Paisano. It's easy to spend hours looking for a place that is within 100 feet of you, and immediately forget how to get back there after you do find it.

But they were finally there. They soaked in the sight of the city as they soaked in the rain. They turned around to ask for more detailed instructions. The water taxi had already sped off and was fading into the distance. Mike and Mary were left standing at the edge of St. Mark's without a clue in which direction to head. The water had started to leak into their suitcases. Mary desperately tugged the zippers together, hoping it would prevent leaking. And Mike couldn't stop grinning.

Why? Because the vacation took place during September 2007. Mike was supposed to be dead by then.

As he puts it, "After some point, you don't let the small things in life bother you."

What do you think of when you hear the word cancer? Is it something that concerns you greatly? Does the possibility of it erupting into your life or the life of a loved one bother you? Perhaps that sounds like a silly question. But there are many dangerous diseases out there and only a few that really occupy the mindset of the public. Sixty years ago smallpox was the embodiment of death. Thirty years ago it was HIV/AIDS. Through it all, cancer has remained relatively resilient to the best efforts of medicine to cure it. For a disease that's been existent from the beginning of time and is so omnipresent it feels as though the general public still doesn't have a good idea of what it really is.

We're going to use Mike's story as an introduction to cancer because his case is unfortunately ordinary. His extended survival is actually the only anomaly in a case that follows the path most people would expect. This story is meant to give an introduction to the basic elements of most cancer cases, so that you're familiar with this world as we plunge into the different themes and questions regarding cancer care we'll see in other people's experiences.

Let's turn back the clock to February 2005. Mike is a self-described iron man and looks the part. "I've been told I look like Jack Lords from Hawaii 5-0," he tells me. I'm not sure who that is but I believe him. In his job as an insurance salesman, Mike can count on one hand the number of days he's missed work. He underwent his yearly physical in which his primary care physician didn't find a single issue. A stress test showed his cardiac health was sublime.

In fact, he was such the picture of health that when he caught a cold and began coughing up phlegm for several days, he quickly made an appointment with his primary care physician. The doctor did a routine physical and noticed a tiny lump near his collarbone. "I'll put you through to an ENT (ear, nose, and throat) specialist to check it out. It might take about ten days to get an appointment," he told Mike.

So right away we have our first question. How is it possible for someone to feel fine and have a cancer growing inside them?

Mary, who worked for a urologist, was worried when Mike told her about the lump. She wanted an immediate opinion on it. She asked Mike to come to her boss's office and had him check it out. The urologist beckoned Mike to open up his collar and began prodding at the tiny lump. "Ten days is too much," he told them.

Mary's employment in the office helped them out at that point. She knew many of the physicians in town, and the connections offered her husband advantages not available to the average person. Her boss spoke to a surgeon he knew, and asked him to do a biopsy right away. Here's our second question: what is a biopsy? There are numerous types of biopsies, but in general all are samplings of body tissues that are then examined under the microscope. Their visual appearance and reactions to various chemical tests allows physicians to identify the type of cancer.

Mike saw the surgeon who put him through another physical examination. He prodded the neck lump and searched Mike's body for other growths. Satisfied that he had not found any others, he inserted a needle into Mike's neck and sucked out tissue.

He collected two more samples. The whole process took five minutes. Within days the results were out.

Mike had cancer.

And this brings us to our third question: what is cancer? Let's answer all three queries right now. To understand the definition of a cancer, you need to know about the microscopic building blocks of the body: cells. It's estimated that the average human body is composed of 50 to 75 trillion cells. At the moment of conception, you start out as one cell. That cell replicates (by dividing into two, then each growing back to full size) into two, those two become four, and so on until the full body is formed. But many cells never stop replicating. Consider blood, for example. It's not as if every time you bleed or donate blood you have less of it permanently. Our body replenishes the blood supply by red blood cell replication. Your hair works in the same fashion. It keeps growing because of cell replication.

Cancer begins when cells in any area of the body start replicating out of control. These cells are abnormal and the body's normal mechanism of shutting down their reproduction is not working. This growth can be infinite. But then what separates a benign tumor from a malignant one? There are certain abnormalities in cells that automatically entail their classification as malignant. This is where a biopsy comes in. The lump in question will have cells sucked out by a syringe or excised from the body in order to be analyzed. The cells are examined visually and chemically to see what changes they have compared to normal cells. This analysis will help determine the type of cancer, prognosis, and treatment.

What is consistent of malignant tumors is that given time they will invade into surrounding tissues and can spread into other parts of the body and then start growing in different organs. This invasion and spread is critical. Benign tumors, on the other hand, do not invade surrounding tissue. This doesn't mean they can't cause harmful effects. For example, a benign tumor inside the throat could keep growing until it causes trouble breathing, but the growth rate tends to be extremely slow and it may take years to grow to a significant size capable of causing harm. It would not be considered a threat to spread to other parts of the body. Once it has been removed it is no longer of any concern. In malignant tumors, it's the uncontrolled growth and invasion of other tissues and the capability to migrate and seed other areas that make these dividing cells dangerous.

When you have a collection of these cancerous cells, at some point in size they become a noticeable lump. This is known as a tumor. It takes over a billion tumor cells to make a mass of one cubic centimeter in size (about one third of an inch). X-rays or even other imaging techniques can't reliably detect masses that small. In fact, at sizes that small they cause no irritation to the body. This is why Mike, by both his own assessment and those used by the medical community, appeared in good health before the tumor showed up. At some point they reach a size where they cause symptoms. But by the time this happens the cancer can be at an advanced stage. So detection at early stages is not easy to do unless you have screening tests for them. At this point we have good screening tests only for a limited number of cancers such as breast, colon, and cervical cancer. For most other cancers, there is no optimal screening test.

Even now, screening tests for lung cancer have not been clearly shown to save lives. The problem is that screening works only if it catches an emerging cancer early enough to change treatment. Remember, the critical point is the spread of the cancer cells. If it hasn't gotten to a point where it has spread, then the management for the cancer becomes easier—all you have to do is remove it. So while there are screening protocols that do help tremendously (breast and cervical cancer come to mind), this is not the case with lung cancer.

All right, so you have a tiny bump inside your body. How could it possibly hurt you? People can die from cancer for a number of reasons. As the cancer cells grow in number they take more and more nutrition away from normal tissue for their own growth. It will act like a parasite. Eventually the patient can succumb because their body tissues deteriorate from the nutrient deprivation, and the growth in the body is dominated by this parasite at the expense of normal tissue. People can also die because the cancer invades space in important areas, for example the brain or the liver. If it invades the lungs, it hampers a person's breathing. In that case, the invasion mechanically interferes with normal breathing. These are just a few of the ways in which cancer can cause damage and eventually death.

Mike had received confirmation of his disease. Next he had to fight it. Within a day, a schedule was made with an oncologist that Mary knew. The oncologist was able to squeeze her husband in as the last patient of the day. The doctor started to fire questions at Mike, all to informally gauge the stage of the disease as well as a baseline of symptoms.

"How long have you known about the lump?"

"Have you been coughing or spitting up blood"?

"Do you have pain in the stomach?"

"Any pain in the bones?"

"Any headaches recently?"

A headache could signal spread to the brain. Pain in the bones or unexplained fractures could mean the cancer had invaded the bones. Mike responded with a quiet "no" to every question except one.

"Do you smoke?" the oncologist asked him.

"Yes."

Mike had been a smoker since he was a teenager. Let's take a moment to examine the effects of smoking with regard to cancer. There are several ways of looking at this. We hear so much about the association between lung cancer and smoking, but how many people who smoke actually end up with a malignancy?

40%? 30%? 25%? Actually (and again, the exact numbers will vary depending on the number of years smoked and the number of cigarettes smoked per day; the rates go up the more you smoke and the longer you have smoked), approximately 17 out of 100 male smokers will get lung cancer. For females, it is less common, with 11 out of 100 being afflicted. It's possible you look at this and still think that the association has been overstated.

Let's look at it another way, though. A non-smoker has a 0.5% chance of dying from a lung cancer by the age of 75. A smoker who quits by age 40 has a 6 percent chance of dying from lung cancer at age 75. Lifelong smoking increases the risk of lung cancer by twenty-three hundred percent in men and thirteen hundred percent in women. These statistics become even more striking when you consider that smokers in general are more likely to get heart attacks, strokes, and other illnesses and injuries. For them to get lung cancer, they have to survive these problems that can kill them earlier, meaning that the likelihood of cancer can be much higher.

The absolute statistic is that over 80% of lung cancer patients are or have been smokers. So yes, smoking matters, and matters greatly.

With that last question out of the way, the oncologist started examining Mike's neck, underarms, and abdomen while looking for additional lumps. He listened to the beat of Mike's heart and thumped on his spine to check for any soreness. Mike remained calm, perhaps to comfort Mary. She was becoming more agitated with every passing minute. She was anxious to start hearing answers to the questions everyone was afraid of. "What's the prognosis?" she finally blurted out. "How are we going to treat him?!"

"Well, I did get the details of the biopsy," the oncologist told them. He delivered the news in an almost monotone voice. Like a stand-up comedian who has to practice his sets over and over to find the right timing and tone, it takes time for a physician to figure out how to deliver awful news to patients. Obviously, an excited or happy tone is out of the question. But a depressed, upset delivery is just as bad. Patients rely on hope and you can't take that away from them. Empathetic neutrality is the key. "You have a type of lung cancer called small cell lung cancer," he told them.

"I thought that was good news," laughs Mike, "small cells had to be less harmful than big cells, right?" Not really. There are two main types of lung cancer: small cell lung cancer and non small-cell lung cancer. The former's name is derived from the fact that the individual cells look small, at least compared to other cells, under the microscope. Unfortunately, despite the name, it tends to be vicious; it grows rapidly and often spreads to other organs early and rapidly. It has a tendency to spread, usually to the brain, liver, and bones.

Let's go back to factors important in cancer: the type and how far it has spread. Finding how much it has invaded the surrounding issues and how much it has spread is called "staging." Staging helps define the extent of the problem and therefore the treatment plan and the prognosis. Small cell lung cancers are divided into two stages: either limited stage disease (where it is localized to one lung *field*) or extensive stage lung cancer (where the disease has spread beyond one lung *field*). It is extremely important to separate these two stages. Extensive stage disease is treatable but not curable; the goal of treatment is to shrink the disease and buy time so quality of life tends to be an important issue. Limited stage disease is treatable and potentially curable, so the goal of treatment is to get rid of the disease completely and therefore the treatment tends to be more aggressive. The biopsy had confirmed only the type of cancer. Now they needed to run more tests to define the stage accurately. What the physicians look for are signs of the cancer beyond the area of the lung.

So they'd need different parts of Mike's body to be visualized clearly. There are several ways to do this, and each scan has its own pros and cons. In this case, a PET scan was ordered.

A PET scan is a test where a sugar is injected into the body. A radioactive substance is attached to the sugar. It lights up on PET scan image. With this we see where the radioactive substances are located in the body. Why would we want to do that? Remember how the cancer cells preferentially take up nutrients compared to normal ones? The idea is that they will do the same with this radioactive sugar. So looking at the scan, you see places in the body that have accumulated more of the radio-labeled sugar, and these areas can be cancer-laden.

Mike's PET scan lit up in the right upper lung and on the left side of the neck as well as in the mediastinum (area in between the two lungs). It didn't show any disease in the liver or bones. This was reasonably good news. Unfortunately, the PET scan does not visualize the brain well. Mike had to get another test: a Magnetic Resonance Image (MRI) of the brain. An MRI is different from other scans, as magnetic rays are used to visualize the brain and can reveal details not seen in a CT scan.

The oncologist called Mike and Mary in for another appointment to discuss the results. "I don't have good news, Mike."

His MRI scan showed a 1-centimeter growth in the left side of his brain.

"You have a lump in the brain—that means you have extensive stage small cell lung cancer." The oncologist told Mike that he needed to start treatment with radiation therapy to the brain as well as chemotherapy right away.

But Mike was hesitant.

"I had just watched a friend go through all of that, and I wanted to delay that punishment for as long as possible," Mike explains. His friend suffered through a year of chemotherapy treatment. Mike figured that all he had gained was an extra month. So he asked his physician how long he would live without any of the treatment. The oncologist was very forthright.

"Mike, on average a person in your situation would have a life expectancy of weeks."

The median survival without treatment for extensive stage small cell lung cancer is twelve to sixteen weeks on average.

Mike still didn't feel anything wrong inside. His cough was a minor irritation. Other than that he felt good. To understand that you have a terminal disease when everything about you screams absolutely normal is not an easy task. And one might suppose, the biggest question is "Why me?"

And that's our next question. We know what cancer is. But why does it happen to certain people? And unfortunately there is no simple answer for this. A variety of components play a part in the development of cancer. One of the most important appears to be genetics.

Pretend I ask you, "Is Michael Jordan genetically blessed?" Your answer is most likely going to be yes. Jordan's height, and his tremendous athleticism, to some extent, are traits he was born with.

What about Albert Einstein? Again, I'm guessing that most people would say yes. He had a talent for physics and mathematics that few will ever possess.

But are the fruits of genetics only limited to talents? What about a man who is a lifelong smoker, lives to the age of ninety, and never gets diagnosed with lung cancer? There are certainly examples of people who lived that life, people who were neither more or less deserving of being afflicted with cancer than their peers. And maybe what separates the fortunate from the unfortunate is dumb luck, courtesy of a genetic code they were born with compounded by stimulants like cigarettes.

Mike's family has a history of cancer. "My dad had cancer in 1971; he was dead within three months," he says. Treatments have improved since then, but the point is that there is a record of aggressive, deadly cancers in his bloodline. We talked about the association of smoking with cancer, and while it does play a major part, it's not enough of an association to say that Mike's cancer is his fault. There are a lot of Mikes out there, puffing away for a long part of their lives, who don't develop cancer.

Even though Mike's physician had painted a dire picture without treatment, Mike was still hesitant to begin. The memories of his friend suffering under chemotherapy were circulating his mind. This is a common reaction, so the oncologist recommended that he get a second opinion. Mike and Mary traveled to University of California, Davis' Medical Center in Sacramento to speak to a lung cancer specialist. The physician offered the same sobering assessment in his appeal to Mike to initiate treatment.

"We deal in numbers. I can't tell you when you're going to die, but if I had a hundred people in front of me in your same predicament, I would say that most would not live past Thanksgiving," said the university specialist.

Mike nodded his head with no flickers of emotion across his face. Was he calm or in shock? Had the reality of the situation settled in? And how did his wife react? "Well, I had to pick up Mary off the floor," Mike laughs.

With such a short predicted life span, the decision was made. Mike returned to his local oncologist to start treatment. It was understood that he had no other reasonable options. This brings us to our next question: How do we treat cancer?

The three main modalities of treatment at this point in time are 1) surgery, 2) radiation, and 3) chemotherapy. Let's examine briefly why each are used, when they aren't used, and issues that come up with them.

One of Mike's first questions was "Why can't I have surgery and just remove everything?" If you can identify a tumor somewhere within a body, you carve out the tissue that contains the tumor and presto, that cancer is gone. But what happens if the tumor has spread? Remember, the critical point of a cancer is when it is has invaded past its original location and seeded into other areas of the body. The surgeons can remove only what they see. So most of the time, if they cut into a person's body, it is with the intent of removing a localized tumor. It's impossible for them to start hunting down cancer cells that have spread elsewhere. So you need a tumor of a visible size in order to have surgery. The location of the tumor is also important. Mike had one in his brain. You can have surgery to remove malignancies inside the head, but it gets difficult, as there are so many vital structures contained within such a small space. Surgery can be fraught with complications, so there has to be a clear benefit before undergoing it.

Then we have radiation therapy. Radiation therapy is the use of high-energy radiation to kill cancer cells by damaging their DNA (think of it almost as an invisible laser). Radiation therapy can damage normal cells as well as cancer cells. Therefore, treatment has to be minimized to only the necessary areas to avoid collateral damage.

And finally there is the option of chemotherapy. Chemotherapy drugs are chemicals injected into a person's blood stream that kill rapidly dividing cells. Remember, that's the defining nature of tumors. But as we mentioned, it is also the characteristic of numerous other cell lines as well. This explains some of the numerous side effects of chemotherapy such as hair loss. Hair cells are always replicating and chemotherapy does not discriminate between the replicating cells that we want to keep around and those we don't. Some of these drugs can be quite harsh and have a lot of side effects and sap a person's energy. So why do we use them? Again, the idea is that if the cancer has spread you have to be able to get rid of all the individual cancer cells. Chemical destruction is the most practical, as these medications can travel to different parts of the body through the bloodstream, seek out cancer cells, and kill them.

"Why can't I get chemotherapy for the brain?" Mike asked his oncologist. Most chemotherapy drugs, in fact most chemicals in general, do not cross into the brain. There is a barrier between the blood and the brain called the Blood-Brain barrier. This is nature's way of protecting the brain from any infections, chemicals, and other bad stuff in the blood. It works well usually, but if for any reason there is an ailment located directly in the brain, then it makes it more difficult to treat the problem. There is also a fear of the ramifications of exposing the brain to harsh chemicals. So for now, radiation is a suitable treatment for targeting a brain tumor.

The treatments required an organized schedule. It was based upon what would be most effective in dealing with his cancer, but also had to give Mike enough time to recuperate from these tiring treatments. Radiation treatment would be given every day for a few minutes. This would last four weeks. The chemotherapy treatment would last for four hours on the first day, and Mike would return one week later for another dose. Then he would get two weeks' rest. This three-week period is called a cycle. Mike was scheduled for a total of six cycles as long as he was responding to the chemotherapy. He was given two drugs called Irinotecan and Carboplatinum. There are more than 100 medications that fit under the chemotherapy category. Each chemotherapy has specific cancers for which it is effective. Some of the medications are well tolerated, and some have significant side effects. For most cancers anywhere from 5-10 drugs are effective. Usually a combination of 2-3 drugs are given initially, followed by others if the initial ones stop working. The names of the drugs aren't important, but what you should know is that 1) there are numerous chemotherapies out there, and 2) only a limited number work for each cancer.

The days before the first chemotherapy infusion were nerve-racking for Mike. Ironically, the image of the worn-out shell of a human stuck in his mind is the effect of the chemotherapy and not the cancer itself. Most people have no idea what the cancer, sans treatment, does to a person.

Mike remembered his first visit into the chemotherapy clinic well. He noted the brown La-Z-Boys strewn about, some facing televisions, and others placed in more secluded corners. Some patients were sitting down with their IV poles next to them. Others were walking, pushing along their poles as they puttered about the room. Some patients even dragged themselves outside for cigarette breaks as they received their chemotherapy. Yes, you can smoke during chemotherapy. Mike continued to smoke, because at this point not smoking wasn't going to miraculously make his disease curable. And with the difficult period ahead, now was not the time to go cold turkey.

Mary's first thought was that the clinic looked like a high school dance, with the men on one side of the room and the women on the other.

Mike, rebel that he was, decided to break the trend and settled down into one of the cushioned chairs beside a pleasant-looking woman. His nurse prepped his IV and began rattling off the side effects of the drugs and what he would feel like. Most importantly, she stressed the need not to panic. With that said, she ran the

IV and hung Mike's drugs onto a pole. The infusion had begun. Mike turned to the woman next to him and introduced himself. She responded by telling Mike her life story—in great, thorough detail. He listened patiently and when she finally paused, he smiled pleasantly, picked up his jacket, and moved to the men's side of the room. He just wanted peace and quiet.

"How will I know that I'm responding to treatment?" he asked the nurse. It wasn't as if he was going to feel an instantaneous change. There are three ways to assess response to treatment. First, are any of the original symptoms alleviated? Second, do the obvious lumps, such as the one perched near Mike's collarbone, shrink in size? Third, do any of the scans show a decreased amount of the cancer throughout the body? Again, the chemotherapy does not work at instantaneous speeds. So these metrics are measured after two to three cycles of treatment. Most important for Mike's situation was how his PET scan would look in a month and a half.

But before any of this happened, Mike changed in ways he didn't want to. Several weeks into his chemotherapy Mike woke up after a great sleep, trudged into his bathroom, and flicked on the lights. He looked the same, but he had bad hair with one patch sticking out to the side. He patted it down and brushed it to the side. The hair parted from his scalp as if it had no roots. He ran his hand through his hair and another patch clung to his fingers.

Mike called for his son, who was startled to see his dad with two giant bald spots. Mike waved it off and handed his son an electric razor. He needed someone to shave his head. Mike had still been feeling relatively the same up until this point. He still had some disbelief about a terminal sentence despite feeling fine.

But if he or anyone else in the family had any doubts about how things had changed, Mike's rapidly transforming appearance were sure to put them at rest.

The side effects of chemotherapy are numerous, and frankly I don't think it does any good to expand on some of the other symptoms Mike had, such as occasional bouts of nausea or heavy fatigue. We're all well aware that these are volatile drugs, but the effects are varied from individual to individual. What is important is how the patient reacts to the process of treatment.

"I began to lose weight, maybe ten, twenty pounds within two weeks," Mike remembers. He was trying to eat healthy, but in the process ended up losing weight. He had given up his late-night cocktails and junk food, especially his favorite snack of gummy bears in the morning. This was not due to any medical advice he was given. In fact his doctors were upset with him for losing so much weight. Radiation and chemotherapy sap your strength more than anything else, and excessive weight loss can exacerbate these problems. But just as with smoking, there was a bigger picture to consider. A healthy lifestyle makes sense if it will improve your life, and helps you live longer. But Mike already had a terminal sentence. Salads and sobriety weren't going to change that. On the other hand his cold turkey from alcohol was emotionally rough and compounding how lousy the treatments made him feel.

"Now is the time to be drinking beer, and eating junk food—but within limits," his oncologist told him, because in the back of his mind, he wanted Mike to enjoy his life while he could.

So Mike resumed his prior diet, now with the goal of gaining back lost weight. The gains were initially slow. He blamed the food industry for making his goal difficult. In maybe the worst excuse since Elin Nordegren rescued Tiger Woods from the back of the SUV with a 9 iron, Mike explained his dilemma: "Have you shopped for peanuts lately? They have low-fat peanuts, and carb friendly peanuts—where have all the high-fat foods gone?" he says.

Mike gave up the alcohol and the junk food, because he figured that's what he was supposed to do when he started receiving treatment. But then why didn't he give up smoking? "That's an interesting question…eh, I don't know," he admits.

The assault from both the therapy and the weight of bearing a terminal disease affected his mental strength. It changed his demeanor. One of Mike's friends, who was also suffering from cancer, gave him important advice during this time. "He told me never lose your attitude and appetite. Don't give in. You can probably lay in bed all day and feel sorry for yourself, but it won't help your strength. I played golf yesterday in a tournament. I hit a ball only 200 yards, not a major accomplishment, but it's something," Mike remembers.

This mental fortitude is not easy to gain. While the physical stress of cancer is already overwhelming, there are the social and mental aspects that are just as harsh. Mike somehow had to prepare himself, family, and friends for his eventual death. It's a job that he feels he botched.

Mike has two sons. At the time of his diagnosis, his older son was beginning a new job, and the younger son had begun a career as a professional golfer. Mike was convinced that his news would disrupt both of them at momentous points in their lives. He didn't want to trouble either of them, so he kept the news a secret. Finally, around early July 2005, friends and family persuaded him to disclose the diagnosis to his children. Mary was especially adamant about it. Whenever either son would call, she would have to pretend everything was fine. Sometimes they would call while he was receiving chemotherapy and she would invent reasons why he wasn't home. It had become too much of a burden.

Mike relented. He invited both children over, sat them down in the living room, and explained his diagnosis. He told them that he had been undergoing chemotherapy and radiation. He told them that his doctors didn't expect him to live much longer. His boys were unhappy, to say the least.

Mike pointed at the corner of the room, where they decorated their Christmas tree every year. "I promise you I will be here in this room come Christmas time, decorating that tree," he told them, though his doctors had not given him an outlook that optimistic. He wasn't lying to them. In the back of his mind he was convinced that his doctors were wrong.

If he could go back would he have done it differently? "Yes, I would have told them sooner," he says. But why didn't he do it in the first place? After a long thought he finally answers. "I thought I was doing them a favor."

Most oncologists feel that hiding the diagnosis and prognosis from loved ones is a bad idea. Eventually, the relatives are going to find out the diagnosis and the outlook.

"I usually have the whole family come in to have a discussion about the treatment plan and prognosis so if any close family member has a question, they can ask the oncologist directly instead of getting second-hand information. When I do this, I also usually get fewer phone calls from anxious family members," Mike's oncologist says.

How much do you think it pained him to not see his children as often as he could? See, Mike wasn't just hurting his children by hiding the news from them. In the fight with cancer, *emotional support is key.* I'd wager it's the reason that so many cancer patients have multiple pets. Mike received a Chihuahua, Hercules, from his stepdaughter shortly after his diagnosis. Between attacking clothes on the kitchen floor and jumping at visitors, Hercules keeps Mike's mind distracted from his problems. More importantly, the dog is energetic. Hercules doesn't know Mike has cancer. He runs around and demands that Mike play with him the same way anyone else does. His interactions with Mike are blessedly normal. That positive social energy is often a counterbalance to the depression that starts to weigh in from the onslaught of changes to a person's "normal" life. That craving for normalcy is what I suspect also might have played a role in his decision to hide the diagnosis from his children.

After two cycles of chemotherapy, Mike had a CT scan of the chest done, which showed that the lung lesions had considerably shrunk in size. He also had an MRI scan of the brain done, which showed that the solitary brain lesion was smaller. It didn't mean he was cured, but it was good news. His disease was responding to the treatment.

In the meantime, his oncologist stressed "quality of life."

"I didn't like that expression at first," Mike says. "It was just too shocking. When he first said that, I began to think that I was going to pass away immediately." After some time though, he began to accept the philosophy.

The treatments went on for four months. The initial response was good to see, but the real test was how everything looked after an entire treatment regimen. Cancers can become quickly resistant to a therapy, and Mike would be in a dire situation if he didn't maintain improvement. It was time for another PET scan. It seemed important for Mike and Mary to review the scan images themselves. By this time they had switched scan centers because it failed their rigorous standards (it had a poor magazine selection). From the lobby they were ushered into a room where the files were on the computer screen. They snuck a peak while waiting for the doctor.

On PET scans, cancer can show up as dark blots or shadows where more of the radioactive sugar has accumulated. The two of them looked for these spots. They almost fainted. There were giant, dark shadows littered across the screen. They frantically pointed them out to the nearest radiology technician, who was walking by. She took one look at the screen and laughed. "Those giant shadows are your gallbladder, your kidneys, and that one on the top is your brain," she explained.

Terrifying. They decided to stop reading the scans themselves. "After a while we stopped looking at them...every time we would be wrong. When we thought they were good, they were actually bad," says Mary. And vice versa. On this occasion, the news was good.

The cancer had regressed. In fact the scan looked normal. Mike was told that he was in complete remission. That didn't mean his disease was cured. Complete remission meant that a clinical examination and scans did not show any visible signs of the disease. The reason it doesn't mean there is a cure is because of the existence of cancer cells that are so small (microscopic) that they aren't visible on any imaging.

Mike figured that at least he had been able to buy a few months. He and Mary celebrated by booking a flight to Maui. The treatments had robbed him of energy in his legs. So for the time being, he enjoyed the island's beauty as Mary pushed him around on a wheelchair. He wasn't permanently debilitated. But after chemotherapy he would be worn out after walking just a short distance.

Chemotherapy's side effects accumulate over time. Mike's strength went first. His patience followed soon after.

"I began snapping at everyone, my kids, my wife, my staff. Over stupid, little things," he remembers. That was at the tail end of the treatment. Why not earlier? Why not right after the diagnosis, or at the beginning of the radiation?

"It wears you down—you think, *Why do I have to go through all of this?*" he explains. Not that he ever thought of giving up, but four straight months of nausea and fatigue (remember also that he handled these treatments better than most other people) had eroded his spirit.

He points to a lamp above his head. "That gave us a lot of trouble." It was an ugly moment, a culmination of all Mike's frustrations boiling over. In the year that followed his diagnosis, he wanted everything that both he and his wife had planned. This included house renovation, and alterations to his will. This all had to be done as soon as possible since he was told he only had up until December.

Back to the lamp story; Mike was very agitated that day. Mary couldn't calm him down. Earlier, Mike had realized that his mood was radically shifting, and asked the doctor what he should do about it. The doctor pulled out his file, and said, "Well, I just met you a few months ago. You're doing well financially, have grown-up kids, you're very healthy, and here I come to pull the rug out from under your feet. I don't blame you."

He continued, "You might benefit from a tranquilizer," and gave him Xanax. It did help calm him down. But on the particular day that he and Mary were setting up the lamp, he hadn't wanted to take it.

Some friends of his were over to help them with the changes they were making in the house. The lamp set-up was proving to be trickier than they expected. As Mike watched his friends play around with it he got inexplicably angry. He lost his temper. "Get the f*$! out!" he screamed. "I don't ever want to see you again!"

Mike's brother had told Mary to give him a call if she ever needed his help. She called him as soon as Mike began his tirade. During this time, another friend arrived and while Mike was shouting, he installed the lamp. On came the lights. Mike paused and took a look at it. "You don't know what the hell you're doing!" he screamed at his friend, an electrical engineer by trade.

But Mike was on the warpath. His frustrations had been slowly creeping up over the past few months as he had sniped at friends, family, and even his work staff. His brother came over, and along with Mary they managed to calm him down to the point that he would take his medication. Crisis averted. Mike would continue dealing with his mercurial mood through the support of his loving wife, kids, friends, and the makers of Xanax.

To reiterate, this was not just the effect of the disease itself, but also a culmination of the changes in his life. For example, Mary says that she quit her job as soon as they got the word that he had only a few months. She was with him 24/7, eating every meal together.

"I treated him like a baby," she admits, and thinking back, she wishes she hadn't. Mike wanted to be normal. When the cancer was in remission he almost felt normal, but all the other signs in his life reminded him that it was abnormal.

Mike's stress also came from unexpected places. Friendly

efforts to help him sometimes didn't have the intended effect. Everybody meant well. They understood Mike's tempestuous emotions. They would stop by and visit, lending that important emotional support. People came to him telling of eccentric remedies that their relatives took when they were ill with cancer. "Everybody means well, but it got to the point where I told Mary that unless they got an alphabet after their name, I'm not listening to them," he laughs (he means MD).

But often, the visits came unexpectedly and Mike couldn't turn down a person who made the effort to visit him. He just wished they would call first, and that he could have more peace and quiet.

As he puts it, "Sometimes they would interrupt nap time, and you just don't mess with nap time." Implicit in that menacing statement is a source of Mike's frustration: lack of time. "We have people over all day, and I would think, *When will we get some time to ourselves*?" he says.

The symptoms continued to pile up. Mike's hand had been numb for several weeks, and he blamed it on his stress. The truth is that every time he had a new complaint, he was afraid the cancer was back. They made a beeline for the oncologist again. The doctor sat Mike down in the examination room and examined his neck and underarm. No enlarged lymph glands were noted. That was a good sign. The heart and lungs sounded normal.

"Do you have any headaches?" he asked. No. "Any nausea or vomiting?" No. "Any weakness of the legs?" No. "Any blurred vision?" No. These questions were important, since headaches and vomiting could be signs of increased pressure in the brain that would indicate the cancer re-growing in that area. The oncologist started a neurological examination.

He had Mike squeeze his hands. Mike was asked to pull the doctor's arms toward him. Mike then had to raise his legs up. These tests determine muscle power in the extremities. Again, if there is a mass in the brain it is likely that it will interfere with some sort of function. The testing did not show any muscle weakness. The right arm remained numb. "We have to do a repeat MRI of the brain," he told Mike, even though he just had one recently. Remember, there is a limit to the size of a mass that every scan can pick up. It was possible that within the time since he received his last MRI and his doctor's visit, a mass had grown to a visible size.

But once again, the news was good. There was no evidence of cancer in the second scan. Incredibly, it turned out Mike had had a stroke, which amazingly enough was good news, because if the cancer had come back and spread to his brain, there would have been few treatment options beyond perhaps more radiation therapy. Fortunately for Mike, his numbness gradually improved and resolved completely. He was advised to take one baby aspirin a day. Often, one small baby aspirin a day can reduce the chances of another stroke. Mike was told to not worry about it. Just go back to his life. But could he stop worrying?

"I think about it every day," he admits. He didn't worry about it so much as it just stayed on his mind. He still felt relatively well and didn't get sick often. But the disease was a label on him, one that people wouldn't stop staring at. His friends and family couldn't pretend he didn't have a terminal illness, and it colored their interactions.

A man at the cancer center told him to go to group therapy sessions where he could express his feelings and share in other people's experiences. Mike didn't want to. He felt that the support of his friends and family had kept him relatively stable. There was no need for him to confide in strangers. That's why he sought out the corners in the chemotherapy clinic, choosing to rest in peace and quiet rather than trade cancer war stories with other patients. But Mary wanted that therapy. It had been hard on her and she was terrified of showing Mike how distraught she really was. Often, she would cry in places like the shower, so he wouldn't see it.

Mike finally agreed to visit a psychologist, but on the condition that Mary went with him. The psychologist had been recommended to them because of her extensive experience with cancer patients.

Mike was less than impressed. "I tell you, she was straight out of Haight-Ashbury," he laughs.

The first thing they noticed as they were invited into the psychologist's office were the bright, multicolored walls. Mike was trying hard to keep a straight face as he introduced himself.

The psychologist started out with a fastball. "How do you see the color blue?" she asked Mike.

He was taken aback. He looked at Mary for help. He got none. "Uh, well it's not brown," he replied sagely. The next hour and a half was dedicated to these philosophical discussions. He and Mary didn't look at each other until they left the office. They knew if they did they would burst out laughing

So did it help? "Hell yes. After we got out of there I said to Mary, this gal is more screwed up than I am," he remembers. Like most other patients, he tried to find humor in his situation as often as possible.

I can't stress the craving for normalcy enough. For people like Mike, one of the greatest desires is to live life in that alternate universe where cancer is a disease that only *other* people have. Even if he tried not to worry about the cancer, he couldn't stop thinking about it because the people around him were constantly worried.

"Most people don't mean ill, but they just say things without thinking it through," as he offers an example. He went to a cocktail party with Mary, and had a great time. A friend walked up to him, and asked "How are you?" Mike reassured him that he was fine. A couple of minutes later he walked away to grab a drink. As soon as he was no longer looking, that friend pulled Mary to the side. "How's he really doing?" he asked. On the way back home, Mary suddenly burst into tears. It's not the sympathy that bothered them, but the fact that their friends had written him off. There were moments where it sounded like Mike had the same thought. "Every time I'm at a unique place, I think will this be the last time I see it?" he muses. Though he was optimistic, and in fact had lasted longer than was expected, he knew at some point the facts of his situation would establish themselves. The incurable disease wouldn't suddenly become curable.

He tried to temper his own hopes by making light of his situation. "Every Christmas, he complains that he shouldn't be here to have to put up all the lights again," Mary jokes.

Two months after being told that he was in complete remission, Mike came down with a fever. What began as a sporadic cough had turned into constant chest heaving that kept him awake throughout the night. He was filling up tissues with thick yellow phlegm. A chest X-ray showed a cavity in the upper part of the right lung. Had the cancer finally come back? A cavity usually signals one of two things: cancer cells eating up a part of the lung, or an area of infection. Sometimes both can happen at the same time.

After several days with fever, an exhausted Mike was brought to the doctor's office. He was ushered into an examination room. The nurse left to retrieve his charts. When she came back, she found Mike lying in the fetal position on the bed. He hadn't slept in days.

Mike was admitted to the hospital and started on antibiotics, but his fever remained recalcitrant. He was entering emergency territory. As they got into his hospital room, Mary saw the first smile on her husband's face in weeks. "What are you so happy about?" she asked him. He told her he was excited because he had never been admitted to a hospital. He figured he would finally be able to get some sleep.

Instead, he was immediately placed into quarantine. Hospitals are very wary about the possibility of tuberculosis. Mike's history of chemotherapy, which weakens the immune system, and the fact that this looked like such a serious lung illness raised some suspicions about it being tuberculosis. When that happens, the first thing the hospital will do is to limit exposure.

"That was like a prison," Mike says. Friends and family that came to visit had to wear masks. Meanwhile, Mike was panicking because he and his brother had coordinated a surprise birthday party for Mary. Finally, on the night before the party, Mike told her about the surprise and begged her to go without him.

"I am not going to have a surprise birthday party for myself, while my husband is lying in the hospital," snapped Mary. It sounds like a small mishap, and maybe it is silly for someone to be agitated about such a thing. After all, it was Mike who claimed he had an epiphany about not being bothered by the small things in life. But look at it from another of Mike's perspectives, one of *lasts*. That could be the *last* time to celebrate a special day with his wife. It could be the *last* time to organize a party.

The scans couldn't elucidate the nature of Mike's ailment. Mike was seen by a lung specialist in the hospital. The physician examined him and determined he needed a bronchoscopy. This is a procedure where a camera is inserted through the mouth and directed down the path of the lungs to look through the airways. This allows the doctor to both physically visualize any mass or infection, and also a chance to take biopsies. Mike's bronchoscopy didn't reveal any masses—and even better, all the samples were negative for cancer.

"So is there definitely no cancer?" Mike asked when told the news. Unfortunately, all the doctors could say was that there were no cancer cells in the specimens taken during bronchoscopy.

What else could cause that kind of a cavity in the lungs? An infection, including tuberculosis or fungus, can cause it. His oncologist explained that because of the chemotherapy, radiation therapy, and underlying cancer his immune system was suppressed. The immune system in a person's body is constantly active, constantly fighting off bacteria, and when it starts to falter, all the numerous amounts of foreign organisms that were being repelled now have open reign to cause trouble. This is a reason why cancer patients are constantly falling sick. Mike was treated with an aggressive dose of intravenous antibiotics. His fever finally broke, he started to feel better, and scans showed that the cavity decreased in size. He was soon released from the hospital.

But for the rest of his life, the cavity never completely cleared. He was told that he would need surgery if he wanted it completely gone, but given his relatively good state of health after the antibiotics and the limited benefits the surgery would provide, he eventually declined.

"Yeah, every so often I cough up blood for a few days, but other than that it's fine," he says to me in the same tone as if he was talking about annual visits to the dentist. He has a new normal. Symptoms that would cause the average person to panic are acceptable to Mike.

Every three months after that, Mike went for a PET scan and a blood test, awaiting the progression of a disease that can't be cured. Is he afraid of those days marked on the calendar? "To be honest, I've gotten used to it." Life returned to normal. He even went back to working.

His scans would show small abnormalities that could potentially be cancerous. But he wouldn't restart the treatment. Why? Wouldn't it make sense to attack the cancer as early as possible? His doctor told him to wait until the changes became larger. That confused Mike. It just didn't make any sense to wait.

But remember, his cancer is incurable. It won't be fully gone if it's treated immediately or far in the future. And the treatments are no walk in the park. As stressed earlier by his physician, quality of life is important. Mike felt good—why change that? Often giving chemotherapy earlier does not change longevity, but interferes with quality of life if the underlying disease is incurable.

He went through more rough patches. It wasn't clear how many of them were directly related to his main illness, but what was clear was that his body was slowly breaking down. While watching golf on the TV one day, he thought to himself that he was enjoying it more than usual. He realized he couldn't hear the announcers. He turned up the volume on his TV. It barely helped, despite the blasting volume. He had no idea how long ago he had lost his hearing.

The second ENT (ear, nose, and throat) specialist he went to (the first one he had problems with—specifically, the physician was too hairy) gave Mike a solution. "You need ear tubes," she told him. It didn't sound too bad to Mike. He recalled that when his boys were six, they had ear tubes. If they could handle it, so could he. Mary remembers it vividly. She had brought him to the clinic and was seated in the waiting room. The way the office was setup, she could see Mike through a window. His face was pale. As the doctor was putting in the tubes he was clutching the arm handles of his chair so tightly his face was losing color.

After all that he had gone through, the ear tubes turned out to be his most painful experience.

"They stick a needle in your ear drum," he explains. Through the needle they injected the tubes so he could hear clearly.

"What was the diagnosis again?" I ask.

"Oh, I had water in my ear."

After the doctor finished, and Mike had let go of the chair long enough to let some blood back to his face he had only one question: How do kids go through that?

"Oh, we knock them out," the doctor chuckled. That would have been more useful to know before the ear torture.

But at least he had his hearing back.

In May 2007, about two years after the initial bout of treatments, the PET scans showed growing masses not only in the mediastinum (central portion of the chest), but also in the rest of his body. Though he was relatively symptom free, that was a dangerous area for the tumor to be growing and would soon cause symptoms due to location and speed of growth. There were two choices: radiation or chemo. Radiation is targeted, whereas chemo affects the entire body. In this case, with only the upper right chest showing multiple lesions, it was felt more reasonable to treat a localized area with radiation rather than chemotherapy. It would have fewer side effects. Further treatment with chemotherapy would be reserved for another day. Once again he was treated with radiation, but this time it was to the chest instead of the brain. Monday through Friday for four weeks, he sat under the radiation therapy machine, and got zapped in the chest for five to ten minutes. The radiation made him tired, but there was no nausea, no vomiting, and no hair loss. A month after the treatment was completed, a PET scan showed that he was in remission again.

This series of events would repeat several months later in November 2007. PET scans at that time would show shadows at multiple sites of the lung, indicating a relapse of cancer. Mike was advised to undergo chemotherapy, because with the estimated size of the cancer nodules, his oncologist guessed that he would start feeling unwell in a short period of time. Mike was despondent. His hair had grown back and he felt fine. He was not keen to restart chemotherapy. Mike's son visited the oncologist in private and told him that Mike had started drinking heavily again. He was also smoking heavily. He would start drinking at 10:00 in the morning and would continue until late afternoon. Given the constant tension in his life, it was understandable.

His quality of life would again deteriorate. His chemotherapy drugs were changed; he was started on Cisplatin and Irinotecan. The treatment continued from November 2007 to March 2008. Repeat PET scans showed dramatic shrinkage of cancer nodules.

Let us pause here just to review how incredible Mike's situation was. For someone estimated to only live several months to a year, a gain of over three years was not just an outlier, it was an absolute statistical rarity. Most patients with small cell lung cancer who have brain metastasis will last much less than one year. In fact, the nature of Mike's cancer was so unusual that between treatments, the oncologist decided to send a biopsy specimen to one of the nearby universities for a second opinion. He was starting to have doubts about the original diagnosis. But the report came back reconfirming that it was indeed small cell lung cancer.

So how did the doctor explain Mike's unusual course of events? "Well, I can just give a statistical average survival rate to patients. There is no way for me to predict how an individual will do with treatment and how long a person can survive. There are always patients who do much better than average. Unfortunately, there are also patients who do worse than average." He quoted a line that he learned from another patient, "Yesterday is history. Today is a gift. Enjoy it. Tomorrow is a mystery."

Mike was first seen by doctors in 2005 and given a median life expectancy of fewer than six months. Three years later, he was still doing well. He had lived to see one son get married and the other engaged. He ignored his prognosis and the lows—all while chugging along. That's a true iron man.

Post Story: In October of 2008, Mike became incoherent and unsteady on his feet. An MRI showed five new shadows in the brain. He received further treatment with gamma knife radiation to the brain. Unfortunately, it was of no benefit. He was hospitalized that month for palliative care. On November 2, 2008 his grandson was born in the same hospital and Mike was able to get a glimpse of the newborn. On November 3, 2008 he passed away, more than three years after he was first seen for an oncology consultation.

"It is unlikely that I will see another case like Mike for the rest of my life. Most patients with extensive stage small cell lung carcinoma live for less than one year. One can give an average life expectancy at the time of diagnosis, but cannot predict survival for an individual," said his oncologist.

Why not?

"Cancers are often treated as one size fits all, but many cancers are individual beasts and can behave differently from the average. This is what gives hope to patients—I may be the outlier."

Marty the Martyr

STOCKTON, CA – At the bustling intersection of Alpine and El Dorado streets, a small billboard rises above the bright green walls of a local car wash. Well, small as far as billboards go. It's still enough to catch the attention of most passers-by who are on the way to St. Joseph's Medical Center or the myriad of clinical offices surrounding it. The hospital purchased the ad space several years ago for its health care campaign to spotlight several sectors of its industry including oncology, cardiology, and pediatrics by showing happy patients. Where most health care ads come across as clunky or frightening (Kaiser Permanente's commercials urging people to "thrive" is straight out of a dystopian horror), these feel relatively normal, perhaps because they feature actual patients and not actors.

Head further south, and at the corner of Pacific and Bianci Streets is a bigger billboard, whose ad space was also leased to the hospital. In fact, all down Highway 99 is a series of billboards temporarily leased to the hospital. And if one were to have passed by any of them from February 2006 through July 2008, they would have seen a strange picture: A middle-aged boxer, who looks a lot like Robert Duvall, laying a haymaker on a punching bag. It's an odd image for a hospital advertisement, but then again, Marty's philosophy is anything but normal.

His story is unique because of his attitude. It may upset some people. I should mention now that it is in no way meant to be disrespectful to anyone afflicted with cancer. After seeing the trauma that cancer patients and their families go through, I wouldn't tell his story if it were. So when I tell you that Marty was excited to get cancer, it does not mean that he is suicidal or mentally deranged. His mindset shouldn't be classified as positive or negative. Marty is a realistic warrior. His refreshingly honest outlook is borne out of respect for his heroes and love of friends and family. In fact, upon knowing him more personally, his approach to cancer seems the only logical fit for his personality.

We're going to examine Marty's story because his attitude is so different. Attitude towards disease is an oft-discussed theme. We've taken it upon ourselves to assume that we have to be positive when dealing with serious ailments. Like any other obstacle, we are told that it is best to face the nadir of life with a smile on our face. Lance Armstrong, the former ambassador of perseverance in the face of cancer, said that one needs to "make an obstacle an opportunity, make a negative a positive." It is taken for granted that there is only one right way to face a terminal condition: the optimistic way. Why? Are there actually attitudes people shouldn't have?

Is it possible, like Marty, to be too positive?

Marty, born and raised in Stockton, CA, has had too much experience with cancer. Out of five uncles and aunts, four have succumbed to the disease. So did his father. His dad, a mechanic, was a stoic, no-nonsense, old-fashioned kind of guy who had been sobered by involvement in World War II. One of Marty's favorite memories was fixing a leaky roof with his father. Midway through the process, Marty saw his dad silently leaving with the nail gun in his hand. He returned a few minutes later and went back to work without saying a word. When he placed a nail into a ceiling board, Marty noticed a bloody bandage wrapped around the index finger.

"What's wrong?" Marty asked his dad. His father told him he had a small mishap with the gun and managed to spike a nail through his finger. He shrugged his shoulders and went back to nailing the roof. Marty slowed down, obviously distracted. His dad noticed. "Is this bothering you?" he asked. "It's just pain. Shut up and go back to work." An embarrassed Marty resumed his hammering.

"It's just pain." That answer sticks with him whenever he's hurting.

In 1996, Marty's father was diagnosed with lung cancer, perhaps as a result of working in a warehouse filled with asbestos during the war. There's a clear link between asbestos and certain lung cancers. Perhaps he would have been afflicted even without working in the warehouse. After all, there is a strong history of cancer in the family. By the time he was diagnosed, he was too far gone to be saved. Days before his father died, Marty held his hand in a musty hospital room. He told him that if he ever had cancer, he would challenge it to the death. Marty had no idea that he had already developed a type of cancer called Non-Hodgkin's Lymphoma.

The signs had been there since January 1995. Itchy skin, rashes, and fatigue, symptoms associated with the disease, had already begun to affect him. He would get a rash for two weeks and then it would disappear. He chalked it up to his work as a landscaper, and assumed that his constant time outside had led to him developing allergies. As for the fatigue, well, anyone working 80 hours a week in the dry heat of California's Central Valley is bound to feel some exhaustion. Marty would ignore these signs, and aside from intermittent bouts of low energy, he would be fine. This continued on and off over months.

Four years later, in December of 1998, he was applying deodorant in his left armpit when he felt a bump. Not being in the habit of looking at his armpits daily, Marty was astonished to see a golf-ball sized lump. Tumors, unlike mosquito bites or skin flare-ups, have a firm to rock hard consistency. That's what it felt like to Marty. Still, he didn't think too much of it. His father's death and the family history of cancer had not made him any more wary of the disease. Fortunately, his first client that Saturday morning happened to be a retired doctor. Marty lifted up his shirt and showed him the lump.

"Get it checked out next Monday or Tuesday at the latest," the physician told him.

Incredibly, Marty still wasn't anxious. However, he decided to go for a second opinion: another doctor client who was on his schedule the following Saturday. He told Marty the same thing. This time Marty got the message and booked an appointment with his primary care physician for the following week.

When a patient comes to a physician with a lump, they are initially examined all over for additional lumps. This is to get a quick, albeit limited, understanding of how far the disease has spread in the event that it is cancer. Though blood work and scans will also be used to identify cancer, every test has its flaws. For example, scans can miss a tumor in the neck that a physician might actually be able to feel with their fingers.

The doctor examined Marty's neck, underarms, groin, then listened to his chest and examined his abdomen. The only finding was the lump in his left axilla (fancy medical terminology for armpit). The next step was to figure out if the lump was benign or malignant.

Two days before Christmas, Marty got a needle biopsy. The biopsy suggested that the aspirated cells were abnormal, but not enough material had been taken out to make a definitive diagnosis. So Marty had another biopsy done where a small chunk of the lump was removed and sent to the pathology team. Marty had set up an appointment for the first week of the New Year to discuss the results. Five days after his second biopsy he got a phone call. The doctor's son, who worked in his dad's office, was on the other line. He asked Marty if he could come to the clinic the next day. Marty knew right away. Urgent news in this case was obviously not good news. He had cancer.

Strangely enough, Marty was pumped.

"It was like an incredible thrill. What an awesome challenge, because I had made this promise to my hero, my dad. It was overwhelming. I did of course realize this could very well kill me," he says. He wasn't ignorant of the complications that lay ahead. After all, Marty had already seen his father, grandfather, and four uncles and aunts die from cancer. And as we'll see later on, Marty's attitude would not change, no matter how pain-free or painful his life was. Marty is a fierce competitor, the type that gets pumped up for even the smallest competitions. To him, cancer was simply the next great challenge. He had told his father that the disease wouldn't intimidate him. In a way, he saw himself as a battleground where physicians could fight this enemy. Marty would put complete trust in his doctors, telling them he would do whatever they recommended. He hoped that he could show other people not to be afraid of the disease without having to put up a façade of optimism.

In an odd way, he was also relieved to know what was actually wrong with him. The sudden fatigue spells and the rashes had convinced him that he was getting too stressed. It was frustrating to have these symptoms that were intermittent and nonspecific. Those kinds of complaints make it difficult for physicians to pinpoint a cause. Knowing the reason behind these complaints was a relief because now he had a goal in his mind and an enemy he could fight. At least, that was his mindset at the time.

"I was actually blessed to get cancer. I know it sounds insane," he chuckles. "It took cancer to change some things in my life. My workaholic behavior, for example." Though perhaps he doesn't intend it, he comes across as being comforted by the fact that his workload was not the source of his problems. Work was his refuge. It would help him keep his mind busy and prevent his obsession over the cancer. His work schedule was a benchmark to measure how severely the disease was affecting him. If his workload was decreasing, it meant that he was really suffering from the symptoms. Single and without children at the time of his diagnosis, landscaping was the major constant in his life. In fact, he considers his journey toward being less dependent on work to occupy his days as a benefit of his fight with cancer.

He phoned his mom to tell her about the doctor's call. Like Marty, she also knew what it meant. She took it hard. She had watched her husband die from lung cancer several years ago. Her dad had also died in 1989 from cancer. Now she faced the prospect of losing her son to the same disease.

"Everything will be fine. I'll be there for you," Marty promised her.

"The way he was supporting me, you would think I was the one with cancer," she laughs.

Marty was told that he had a type of cancer called Non-Hodgkin's Lymphoma (NHL, not to be confused with the even less-popular National Hockey League). NHL is not a common cancer. It constitutes only 4% of all newly diagnosed cancers. Around 65,000 new cases of Non-Hodgkin's Lymphoma are diagnosed each year in the United States. The chance of developing Non-Hodgkin's Lymphoma is one in fifty, or 2% in your lifetime. The number might sound high, but notice the word "lifetime," which is different from saying 2% of people will develop the disease.

Lymphomas are somewhat different than the cancers you are used to hearing about such as colon cancer or lung cancer. To fully explain it we're going to have to go through a lot of jargon, so I'll spend a little time breaking it down before we get back to Marty. This will also help us understand what Marty was about to go through and the severity of his disease. A lymphoma is a malignant growth that arises from lymphoid tissue. Lymphoid tissue is present in many different sites in the body. It is associated with the body's immune system, either producing or regulating it. Marty discovered the tumor in his armpit because there are many lymph glands in that area and one happened to gather enough of the tumor cells so it enlarged. The other main lymph glands are found in the neck, groin, chest, abdomen, and pelvis, and those are also common sites of involvement with lymphoma.

For the vast majority of NHL, no cause is known. There are associations with different diseases including lupus and HIV, but the vast majority of cases (including Marty's) have none of the associated illnesses.

Once NHL is diagnosed, the next step is to confirm and define the type of NHL. There are nearly fifty different types of NHL and the outlook and treatment can be very different depending on the type of lymphoma. So, defining the type of lymphoma is critical to defining the treatment plan and prognosis. Often the biopsy sample is sent to a major university center, where special studies are done on the specimen and a pathologist who specializes in these types of tumors can examine it. In Marty's case the biopsy specimen was sent to Stanford University. The results came back from Stanford showing a type of lymphoma called Follicular Lymphoma. This was critical information, because Follicular Lymphomas are usually considered low-grade. For practical purposes, NHLs are divided into low-grade lymphomas and high-grade lymphomas. Low-grade lymphomas tend to grow slowly and patients can live with them for many years without needing treatment. We'll go into detail on the reason for that in a bit. High-grade lymphomas, on the other hand, tend to evolve and grow quickly, and unless treated appropriately and aggressively, can be rapidly fatal.

The next task is to stage the disease. The purpose of staging is to define the extent of the cancer. Doctors have to determine whether the disease is limited or more advanced and widespread. Staging of lymphomas is analyzed through an assortment of procedures that include blood tests, CT scans of the chest, abdomen and pelvis, PET scans, as well as biopsies of the patient's bone marrow.

As you will see for all cancers, lower numbers indicate a more benign stage. For lymphomas, Stage I means the disease is localized to one area. Stage II is disease in two or more locations on the same side of the diaphragm. Stage III is disease on both sides of the diaphragm. Stage IV is when a major organ such as the lungs, liver, or bones and bone marrow is involved (this is a general description, and certain rare cases can circumvent this staging). This might sound odd since most cancers that people are familiar with already involve an organ, such as lung cancer or liver cancer. But remember, a lymphoma is a *blood* cancer, as the cancer arises from cells that exist in the blood, and so the staging criteria is different than for organ malignancies.

Marty's bone marrow biopsy, performed four weeks after his diagnosis, showed involvement with lymphoma. Therefore, Marty had stage IV Non-Hodgkin's Lymphoma. Though it indicates the widest spread form of the cancer, it is actually a common diagnosis. Roughly 90% of people with Non-Hodgkin's Lymphoma at the time of initial diagnosis are either stage III or IV.

One last way to describe a lymphoma is to categorize it by the symptoms that it causes. In NHL there can be three common complaints: unexplained weight loss of more than 10% of a person's baseline weight; drenching night sweats; and persistent fevers. If you have any of these complaints, then the suffix B is added to the stage. For example, Stage III with these symptoms will be called Stage III B. Without them, it will be known as Stage III A. B symptoms (as they are called) are thought to be related to volume of disease. While Marty had been fatigued and itchy for some time, he had none of the three B symptoms. His final diagnosis then was Stage IV A Follicular Lymphoma.

Whew! That was a lot, right? But it was important for his physicians, because it allowed them to figure out his treatment plan.

This plan includes the vital question of when to start treatment.

Everyone assumes that treatments begin immediately, but that isn't the case. The best way to understand this is by examining goals. Physicians usually have two goals for a patient. First, they want to know if the disease can be cured. Cure means the disease never ever comes back and the patient continues their natural life span without any evidence of the disease on any type of examination (clinical examination, blood work, or any X-rays or scans). At this point in time, the accepted stance is that low-grade NHL, at Stage III or IV, is incurable. That isn't exactly true, as there is the chance of a cure through an allogeneic stem cell transplant (bone marrow transplant), which we will discuss later. However, it is seen as a last-ditch effort because the process is so incredibly risky. Interestingly, high-grade NHL has almost a 60% cure rate even though it is more aggressive. In the rare case that a Stage I or Stage II low-grade NHL is discovered, radiation alone cures about half the cases.

The second goal, ascertained if the disease is not curable, is to make the person either feel better and/or live longer. The goal therefore is to treat symptoms and reduce the pain and discomfort that the patient may be suffering. The issue with low-grade Non-Hodgkin's Lymphoma is tied into its slow-growing nature. It can take years for it to grow to a fatal volume within the body. You're probably thinking that is a good thing. It is, but it also creates the interesting dilemma of when to treat the disease. The conventional wisdom with any disease is the earlier it gets treated, the better. That certainly makes sense if the disease is curable. What if it isn't? In that case, the attention shifts to the second goal. With low grade Non-Hodgkin's Lymphoma, the ideal approach is to start treatment when symptoms arise and the disease is interfering with daily activities. Early and aggressive treatment will not prolong life, but it does interfere with quality of life, as the patient now has to deal with side effects of treatments like chemotherapy, which we know can be quite significant.

For example, pretend you discover a lump in your neck and a lump in your groin and a biopsy reveals a low-grade Non Hodgkin's Lymphoma. Let's also pretend that the average life expectancy with this form of NHL is ten years. But you have no complaints. You don't have the itching or the fatigue or the night sweats. But you're still nervous. You want to be proactive in attacking the disease. You then look at the options available.

There are three of them: radiation therapy, medications (chemotherapy), or monitoring your health without any active treatment. Radiation is very effective, but it helps shrink disease in only a localized area (the area being treated). It has no effect on areas not covered in the radiation field. Because they are blood cancers, lymphomas are usually a systemic disease. Therefore, it would not be practical to give radiation therapy. In order to kill all the lymphoma cells you would have to irradiate the entire person, head to toe. That would cause severe damage and significant side effects, and certainly not be pragmatic. The next available option is the pharmaceutical approach. Via the blood stream, chemotherapy will target the cancer all over the body. If you remember in Mike's story, chemotherapy is medicine that targets rapidly dividing cells. The problem, though, is that chemotherapy can often have harsh side effects, including fatigue, hair loss, and in many cases strong nausea. Okay, so you're still willing to pay that price, even though you feel fine right now. You go through chemotherapy. On the scans, you look at the tumors and measure how they shrink after treatment. You can no longer see these tumors on the scans! The tumor went away! You feel good about your decision even though you're now bald, nauseated, and constantly fatigued.

Success, right?! Yes and no. The visible tumors may have disappeared on the scans. But there are still cancer cells left behind which are too small for imaging to visualize. For reasons unknown at this point, in a low-grade lymphoma there are always cancer cells resistant to the chemotherapy. It is why the disease is considered incurable. What you've achieved is an X-ray, CT scan, and PET scan success, not a cure. So now you have to deal with the side effects of chemotherapy, and although the tumors shrank, they will almost surely return. Your life expectancy has not changed. In fact the only thing you've done is to make yourself feel worse by subjecting yourself to the side effects of treatment with no change in longevity.

It's difficult for many people to wrap their minds around the concept of delay and medical pacifism. Many physicians have difficulty convincing their patients to "do nothing." In this age of proactive attitude, restraint is an elusive virtue. Marty would have had little problem with this plan. His full, almost blind faith in his physicians let him follow their recommendations obediently. However, as we saw earlier he had already been suffering from pain, rashes, and fatigue. This was indication to start treatment in order to alleviate the symptoms and improve the quality of his life.

After his diagnosis, Marty discussed treatment options with his oncologist. He was prescribed a chemotherapy medicine called Chlorambucil along with Prednisone, which is a type of steroid. Both are in pill form, so Marty did not require intravenous treatments. These drugs were chosen because they are usually very effective in controlling the disease without too many side effects. Marty was also sent to Stanford University for another opinion. He was sent there more for reassurance, as the treatment was fairly standard, and to confirm the plan. Stanford University physicians reviewed all the information including the pathology, X-rays, and the blood work. His Stanford healthcare providers agreed with the plan and made no modifications. So Marty continued these medications for several weeks between March and July of 1999.

Meanwhile, he kept his day job. Not only that, but he increased his working hours. In the dry summer heat of Northern California's Central Valley, he maintained gardens and yards at a 90-hour per week schedule.

Why on earth did he do this? It's not as if the chemotherapy wasn't having effects. The prednisone began to cause Viagra-like effects. Marty responded by wearing extra-large sweatshirts. Of course, wearing heavy layered clothing while working outside in the summer created its own problems. The extra warmth fatigued him even faster. His schedule was to receive the treatment for five straight days every four weeks. On the days off (from the treatment, not from work) he would be completely drained of energy. It culminated one morning when a client found him standing on a lawn leaning on the handle of his lawnmower, fast asleep. Several times, he would become nauseated and vomit in the bushes. There was concern that this breakneck work pace was harmful. But Marty had checked with his oncologist beforehand about continuing to work. He was told that pushing himself would not interfere with the efficacy of his treatment. Nor would rest improve the treatments. But family and friends, especially his mother, were very worried as they watched Marty push his limits.

After three months of chemotherapy his scans were again

repeated. There was no evidence that the disease had regressed. Although Marty tolerated the oral chemotherapy well, he continued to feel tired. He was then started on second line chemotherapy, which meant that the drugs were changed. (There are multiple chemotherapy drugs that are used against lymphoma. They are often effective, but not always. The only way to find out is to try them out. The principle is to use a combination of 2-3 drugs at a time to see if they work. Usually treatment is given for 2-3 months and if effective, it is continued for 4-6 months. There is no other way to predict if the drugs are going to help. Usually the most effective combination with the fewest toxic side effects is used initially. Drugs with more serious toxicity are used down the line.) He received two chemotherapy drugs given intravenously, called Cytoxan and Vincristine, as well as Prednisone again by mouth. (This is referred to as CVP. Oncology drugs are frequently cocktails of medicines and these acronyms are used to describe different combinations). He received five cycles of this treatment (each cycle consisted of one treatment every three weeks) from September to December of 1999. This time, the tumor in the left underarm shrank partially. The success was short-lived, because after the treatments stopped the disease began to progress again. Chemotherapy can't be continued forever, so you want the drugs that are used to be effective.

He was started on third line treatment in the form of a relatively new drug called Rituximab (Rituxan). It was part of a new class of drugs referred to as target-specific drugs. They attach specifically to targets on the lymphoma cells and kill them. Since they are target-specific, the side effects tend to be fewer, so there are none of the common side effects of chemotherapy like vomiting, hair loss, or low blood counts. But even the drugs that look good on paper can still cause issues, as Marty soon found out.

He was started on Rituxan in November 2000. Two hours into the first infusion, Marty began to wheeze and shiver violently. "I felt really cold all of a sudden. It wasn't that I was just shivering uncontrollably. It was as if the temperature in the room had plunged," he remembers. "I tried to relax and then I felt my teeth start to chatter."

Marty raised his shaking hands, calmly asking for help from a nurse. "I didn't panic...the nurses were there. It's their responsibility to fix it and panic," he shrugs. And in fact such a reaction is not a major issue; although the symptoms can be quite severe, they are not usually life-threatening. It's not an allergic reaction, but more of an adjustment to the drug by the body. He was given some oxygen, covered with blankets, and Rituxan was discontinued for a short while. Thirty minutes later they began the treatment again and the dose was increased slowly. This time there were no further reactions. If you're wondering why they even continued with Rituxan, it is because the side effect itself is not indicative of a treatment not being right for the patient. It just means there needs to be an adjustment phase.

Days later, as he was about to take a shower he noticed a long rash running across his back and chest. It was filled with tiny red bumps. Some were filled with specks of yellow fluid, pus. He gingerly touched one and winced in pain.

He had developed Shingles. Shingles is also known as herpes zoster. This is a complication of lymphoma that occurs in almost 100% of lymphoma patients during their lifetime. Herpes Zoster, also called varicella, is the same virus as the chicken pox virus. Most human beings carry the virus forever if they have had chicken pox. The virus tends to reside dormant in nerve endings.

Anytime the body's immune system is stressed, the virus can flare up in the form of a painful rash in the path of different nerve endings. It can be treated but cannot be eradicated.

The rash lasts for about a week and then gradually dissipates. It tends to be only on one side of the body and it rarely crosses the midline. In Marty's case it was on his right side. "It felt like the skin was burning. Ice packs didn't really help. I finally just ignored them." Marty used the silent treatment to great effect, and it worked as well on shingles as it does on most men. After all, it's just pain.

To help him though, he was given standard antiviral drugs. The rash gradually disappeared and the pain went away, although not fully. Shingles usually leads to permanent discoloration at the sites of the rash and patients can have discomfort and pain for years there. Even after the blisters went away, it was painful for him.

Marty actually felt at home in the infusion room. Maybe it was because he treated it like a rest stop. Sometimes he would landscape in the early morning, finish several hours of work, and then come to the clinic to receive his Rituxan infusion for a few hours.

"Do you have a ride back home?" a nurse asked him in one of his early sessions.

"Nope, I have a ride back to work," Marty replied enthusiastically. Most of the time he would nap while receiving treatment, but occasionally people wanted to talk and get perspective about their own battles. Having cancer puts you in an exclusive club, one that no one wants to be a part of, but whose members immediately begin to relate to one another.

I often wonder what went through Marty's mind, looking at

the other people who go through the same battle but with the polar opposite mindset. As hard as it is for most people to understand his attitude, does he have the same difficulty putting himself in the shoes of those who wilt away in the face of cancer?

Marty wants to be a martyr for cancer. Don't confuse that with a desire to die from the disease. His interest is in pushing onward, and not letting the cancer dominate his life in any way. "I felt that as long as the vital organs, such as the heart and lungs, were strong I would be fine. If all I had to suffer was fatigue and pain, then I could deal with it. To that end, I never asked for an expected survival time," he says.

Statistics did not matter to him. How would knowing a due date for death help him? He would approach life the same way whether he was going to die in five years, ten years, or fifty years. All he knew was that his cancer was a low-grade lymphoma. That meant that it would be slow-growing, and that meant he had years to live.

In February of 2000, almost a year and half after his diagnosis, he developed severe pain in his joints. He first experienced it in his shoulder. It felt like arthritis. Some of the joints were swollen and stiff, making it difficult to move. Marty had to start using a walker. "Every day, I would look at my knees or wrist, some days it was my ankle and elbows, and I could see them getting larger. My knees literally doubled in size from the swelling," he remembers. The swelling would fluctuate quickly, too.

One day he was mowing a client's lawn. When he arrived to the house that morning he had not been in too much pain. As he pushed around the lawnmower, he noticed it was getting more difficult to maneuver. He looked at his wrists. They were engorged. Soon, it was painful for him to even rest his hands on the lawnmower handles. He had a job to do, though, and he was going to finish mowing the lawn. But that would not be the most difficult part of his day; he also had to load the machine into the back of his truck and drive back. He stood in the lawn, and looked at the equipment as he thought, *How am I going to get home?*

How did he do it? "I just thought of my dad," he explains.

At first, his doctors were concerned about the possibility of gout, which can sometimes occur in multiple joints in patients on chemotherapy. They quickly discovered it wasn't gout. X-rays and other scans did not show any evidence of joint damage. What the scans did show were changes suggesting that it was actually the lymphoma, which was infiltrating his bones, making them fragile and painful. This was unusual. Typically, lymphomas do not affect the bones so dramatically. He was prescribed anti-inflammatory medications like ibuprofen as well as narcotics for pain control. Despite taking these medicines, he continued to have significant pain. Keep in mind that he was still receiving chemotherapy. Soon Marty would often head to the hospital for pain control, starting in September of 2001. Every two to four months for the next two years he would be admitted for intense pain. Pain management was basically a series of narcotic painkillers that were slowly increased in potency until he could manage with non-IV medication. But when he could walk freely, he was still doing his landscaping. He even asked the doctors for an intravenous narcotic pain medication backpack so he could do his work while receiving treatment. His request was of course denied. His physicians didn't think it would be a good idea to work while having narcotics pumped intravenously through his system.

In August 2001, he had another scan. The mass in the left

axilla (armpit) now measured 7.5 cm. He also had developed a mass in the left supraclavicular region (above the clavicle) that was 3.5 cm. The disease was slowly progressing.

Often the pain and aching got so bad that he couldn't sleep. Eventually, the pain and inflammation moved up into his face. Early in 2002, Marty woke up one morning without vision in the right eye. His right cheekbone had actually swollen up so much that it blocked his eyeball. He felt his face. The skin was smooth, glass-like, sort of as if it had been burnt. A CT scan revealed that the cancer was invading the tissue there. When lymphoma gets into the bone marrow (the pulp in the center of bones) it can spread throughout the entire skeletal structure. Thus, even the cheekbones are fair game for this invader. In these instances, there really isn't much the doctors can do outside of giving narcotics for pain. Radiation therapy can sometimes be used to treat significant areas of pain.

There is, at the moment, no understanding of why the cancer invades peculiar areas such as the right cheekbone but not the left one as in Marty's case. Marty tried ice packs for the swelling, but it didn't help. All he could do was wait. Two weeks later the swelling went away, but the doctors told him that it could swell up in the other cheek just as easily. The next week Marty woke up with his left eye blocked by the swelling. Again, all he could do was wait.

Marty still continued to work throughout this. After all, it wasn't like both eyes were covered. "When you do gardening, everything is so repetitious, you could do it blindfolded, so the lack of eyesight didn't bother me," he explains. He wore goggles to hide the swelling, but it's somewhat difficult to hide the fact that half your face is puffing outwards. One concerned client asked about the swelling. Marty, paused before replying, "The truth is, I had a date last night and it didn't go so well...."

After four years of treatments, he had still not beaten back the disease. To put it another way, Marty could have received no treatments at all in the past four years and would still be in the same situation, save for the temporary relief of some symptoms. So why even go through any of the chemotherapy, radiation, etc.?

Unfortunately, doctors have difficulty in predicting how quickly or slowly the disease will progress and for how long a person will survive, especially in low-grade Non Hodgkins Lymphoma, as the rate of progression can vary tremendously from individual to individual. These difficulties also apply to treatment. Different chemotherapy combinations can be tried, but it is difficult to predict if a treatment cocktail will work, how well it will work, and if it does work how long will it work. In Marty's case it was very obvious the disease was slowly but relentlessly progressing. It was also obvious that in the near future Marty would be in deep trouble as the amount of lymphoma in his body steadily increased. Since conventional chemotherapies were not working, Marty, after discussion with his oncologist, got in touch with Stanford to participate in clinical trials. The advantages were very clear to him. First, he might receive treatment that could actually cause regression of the cancer. Second, he wanted to be a guinea pig for medicine. Even if he didn't benefit from the research, others would. "I would be honored to be part of the progress made in fighting cancer," he explains.

In 2002, Stanford notified him that he was a candidate for a clinical trial. Doctors were attempting a type of injectable radiation called Zevalin. The principle of this treatment is that a radioactive isotope is attached to a protein, and in turn the protein has the capability of attaching specifically to lymphoma cells so radiation therapy is given directly to lymphoma cells with very little collateral damage. Simple, right? (Just nod your head and keep reading.)

The physicians wanted to test his heart and lungs to see if he was strong enough for their trial. It was an exciting prospect for Marty until he got a call saying the trial had been postponed. The Food and Drug Administration (FDA) wanted to collect more data on several patients before giving re-approval to continue the trial. Marty would wait even as he and his doctors saw little promise in other standard treatments (Zevalin has now been approved by the FDA for use in treatment of lymphomas).

At the same time, his doctors were considering a stem cell transplant, a last-ditch effort for treatment of lymphomas. Feeling that he could go back to the clinical trials if the prospects of a stem cell transplant did not look good, Marty agreed and they began to look for a match.

So how do stem cell transplants work?

Remember how we've talked about the limitations on the amount of chemotherapy you can give? The idea behind the transplant is to get rid of dose limitations. The patient will receive very high doses of chemotherapy and perhaps radiation therapy. The hope is that such high doses will eradicate any and all cancer cells in the body. But when this is done, it also wipes out all the cells in a person's bone marrow. The bone marrow is the organ that produces all the blood in the human body (red cells, white cells, and platelets). After high dose treatments, the contents of the bone marrow are wiped out completely so that no further blood is being produced. If you stop at this point, the patient will die. This is where the transplant comes in. After administration of the high dose chemotherapy, bone marrow cells are infused intravenously into the patient. These stem cells migrate and lodge in the empty bone marrow spaces and start producing blood again. There are two common sources of bone marrow donors. If the bone marrow is collected from the patient himself/herself prior to high dose chemotherapy, then this is termed autologous stem cell or bone marrow transplant. The process of collecting stem cells is called bone marrow harvesting. If the bone marrow cells are collected from another human being it is called an allogeneic transplant. Allogeneic transplants are usually more effective than autologous transplants at curing the cancer, but they tend to have a much higher mortality and morbidity rate. I'll explain why later. In Marty's type of lymphoma, autologous transplants are not usually successful, so an allogeneic transplant was recommended.

The first place to look for a bone marrow match is immediate family. Not the mother and father, because they will never be a full match, but brothers and sisters (basic biology. Your mother and father each provide half of your DNA, so they can only be a 3 out of 6 match). They tested Marty's brother, but he was not a match. So they put Marty on an international watch list. There is a 1 in 20,000 chance of finding a perfect match for the transplant. Of course Marty was amped when he was told about this. For him, those were great odds. "With a 1 in 20,000 chance, I'm thinking great because these odds begin with a 1," he says. In the meantime, he was free to go back to the clinical trials. By this time the FDA had given Stanford approval again for the Zevalin trial, but they had run out of room for him after collecting the twelve patients they needed. Once again, Marty watched another opportunity slip through his fingers.

While awaiting the results of the donor list, Marty's disease relentlessly worsened. His complaints increased. His joint pains continued.

One of the biggest problems with joint pain was the fatigue. Dealing with extreme pain is tiring. Couple that with the fact that it was preventing Marty from getting sleep and he was having a hard time keeping up with his 90-hour work week.

It was time for sacrifices. Marty cut his workload to an 80-hour week and sometimes even only 70 hours. As he fell behind in his work schedule, his nephew chipped in to keep the business from suffering.

Further chemotherapy drugs were tried, including Mitoxantrone, Fludaribine (MF), and Cytoxan, Prednisone, Etoposide, Procarbazine (CEPP). But just like the rest of the conventional treatments tried so far, these were, at best, of minor benefit to him. During a particularly painful episode, he had X-rays of the left knee and femur done. These were normal, but an MRI of the left knee and ankle showed that his bone marrow was heavily infiltrated by lymphoma. He received radiation therapy to these affected bone areas for pain control alongside the narcotics that he was already on. Marty was now entering dangerous territory.

In November 2003, Marty was readmitted to the hospital to start a more intensive chemotherapy regimen that consisted of Rituxan-Etoposide, Cisplatinum, Cytarabine, and Methylprednisolone (R-ESHAP Protocol). This was another cocktail of chemotherapy drugs, but one in which Marty required admission to hospital for an expected four days in a row (admission is required for this combination of chemotherapy drugs as these medicines have to be given in 12 to 24 hour continuous infusions along with large amount of fluids, so outpatient administration can be very difficult). Because of the significant side effects, though, his hospital stay usually ended up being five to six days. This continued on a monthly basis for six cycles of treatment, until April of 2004. You should notice that as the disease progressed, not only did its effects on Marty increase in severity, but so did the side effects from the treatments. As both the patient and the physician became more desperate to turn the tide, the treatments they relied on came at higher costs in terms of quality of life.

After the third treatment, Marty decided to attend a medical symposium on lymphomas. One of the keynote speakers was his clinical supervisor from Stanford. After her speech, Marty surprised her backstage to show her how well he was holding up. She was amazed at his good condition and recommended that he continue on for another two treatments after the initial six. However, this concept of "good health" has to be kept in perspective. Marty was holding up well compared to others who had undergone the same regimen. But he was completely drained. He vomited often, and needed frequent naps throughout the day. He pushed his body, but despite his will, it would not respond adequately. By the end of the sixth treatment, he was in no shape to do two more cycles. The new intensive chemotherapy achieved what nothing else could: Marty had to give up his gardening.

He sent the following letter to all his customers:

"It brings me much pain to write this letter to you. I regret to inform you that my cancer has progressed to a point where I need to take immediate action. I will be retiring from gardening. As of November, my Gardening business will be taken over by my nephew Steven. I am confident that your level of service will remain the same. I would like to thank all of you for your loyalty, kind thoughts, and prayers."

He would not return to his work as a landscaper.

But something wonderful happened with the new regimen. The disease began to shrink and despite the fatigue and vomiting with the chemotherapy, this was wonderful news for Marty. His bone pain improved tremendously. He was popping less pain medications. However, his physicians were still concerned. They knew that despite the good response to these different chemotherapy agents, the effect would not last very long and the disease would certainly grow back in the near future.

Stanford had been looking at the transplant list for a while, but could not find a perfect match. A match is based on something called HLA testing (Human Leukocyte Antigen). Human leukocyte antigens are proteins found in most cells in our body. Our system uses these proteins as markers to recognize which cells belong in our body and which do not. Think of them almost as pieces of uniform for the cells in your body. A 6 out of 6 match is the same uniform, a 5 out of 6 match means you're wearing different boots, and a 1 out of 6 match means one side is wearing a green uniform and the other has on neon orange clothes. If your donor's HLAs are different from yours, your body will recognize them as being foreign and attack these cells, leading to potentially significant side effects. A close HLA match will decrease the chances of such a reaction. The number of HLAs of donors and recipients that are tested in a match are usually 6.

What Marty did not know is that Stanford had found a 5 out of 6 match, from a donor in Germany. They had been waiting for a perfect match, but finally Stanford decided to go forward with it. They had had success with that level of match before. Marty received the call in the middle of June 2004, a month and a half after the intensive chemotherapy treatments had ended.

They gave Marty five weeks to prepare. This meant that he had five weeks to get his life on track, because the transplant process alone puts you out of commission for three to six months. However, there's also the risk of the procedure to consider. The mortality of the transplant is extremely high. The odds were not with Marty.

Of course, a 5 out of 6 match does not give the highest chance of success, but Marty's options were limited. In fact there were no other reasonable options. Marty had agreed to do whatever the doctors felt was best. They had wanted a perfect match, but with so much wear and tear on his body over the past five and a half years, they figured that they needed to take advantage of this opportunity as the disease had shrunk dramatically with the present chemotherapy. The less disease there is, the better transplants work. Marty's recent success with chemotherapy had landed him in the sweet spot for transplants. This transplant would be conducted in a new way. A drug was going to be given before the transplant and evidence behind it suggested that it could limit negative immune responses in the host. Marty's treatment plan would get featured in a multitude of publications, including the *New England Journal of Medicine*.

With a transplant, there are no guarantees of success. You'll see what I mean shortly. One can die from the transplant or have significant morbidity. Marty was clearly aware of the potential pitfalls of his treatment. Before his transplant, he worked out the full transaction of his landscaping business to his nephew. Whereas earlier he had made the handover temporary, the implications of his upcoming treatment meant that he had to stop the work permanently. His blood counts were too erratic, and sometimes his platelet levels (responsible for clotting blood) were dangerously low. Our bodies are constantly plugging up wounds; we just don't notice until we have a deficiency in something as vital as platelets. Marty would be working in a rose bush and barely brush his calf onto a rose thorn. The small prick would cause a bleed that couldn't be stopped. It simply wasn't reasonable for him to work, either at that point or in his near future.

The transplant was scheduled on July 30, 2004. Marty checked into the hospital on July 18th. Before a transplant begins, there is a preparatory period in order to weaken the body's immune system. The human body is naturally wired to reject foreign substances. This inherent defense mechanism makes transplants tricky. For example, our blood is categorized into 4 sub-types (A, B, AB, and O). Depending on your blood type, the body may recognize another person's blood as foreign and begin to destroy it, harming you in the process. The same principle applies to the HLA system. Even with a 6/6 match in a bone marrow transplant, there is still a possibility of the body recognizing it as foreign. So the only potential way to get by this issue is to actually weaken the body's immune defense mechanisms so that it cannot attack the foreign bone marrow. This allows for the transplant, but it also makes you vulnerable to infections and diseases that the body's immune system would normally fight off.

Marty was admitted on a Sunday night. As he checked into his room, he noticed the patient just across the hall from him. Marie, 28 years old, was also set to receive a transplant. The two of them began talking as they pushed their IV poles to the radiology section to get a chest X-ray. She introduced him to her dad, mother, and brother. Marie had already undergone an autologous transplant a year earlier using her own stem cells. When that did not work, they decided to use the half match from her father. It wasn't ideal, but at least there was hope. Marty wished her luck. He felt bad, but had his own battle to go through.

On Monday afternoon, at 1:00, the nursing staff began infusing Anti-Thymocyte Globulin (ATG). The official description of ATG is that it is horse or rabbit derived antibodies that reduce immune competence in people with normal immune systems. (I know you don't know what that means. Heck, I don't know what that means.) In practical terms though, it weakens your immune system. It was done to help prevent rejection of the donor's bone marrow by Marty's body.

Three hours into the infusion, Marty's mom told him she was leaving the hospital. She didn't have a place nearby to stay that night, and so she was headed to her sister-in-law's house, half an hour away in Los Altos. Satisfied that everything was going smoothly, she said bye to her son. Soon, Marty began to feel a pain in his hip. What began as a tingle soon was a burst of pain that shot down his right leg. He could actually feel his own heart rate becoming irregular. His body quivered and his breathing became more difficult. His blood pressure, being monitored closely, went haywire. Five hours into the infusion he was vomiting so forcefully that his gut was becoming sore. Sweat poured from everywhere on his body.

Marty thought, *This could very well be the end.* But he was at peace with that outcome. If it was the end, then what a fight. The pain might have been severe, but he never felt suicidal or desperate. "I was thankful my mom had left, so she didn't have to see me like this." Fortunately, he survived.

Marty considers the ATG to be the second worst pain he ever felt. Since he's dealt with pain so well in the past, how does he react when the pain overruns his mental defenses? "I think about how my dad taught me to endure physical pain, not to back down from it. When it got too severe, when I couldn't handle it, I gave it all to God. There was nothing more emotionally and physically I could give. Spiritually I was still strong though," he tells me.

The ATG continued from the 19th to the 23rd of June. He subsequently had the weekend off. But during the same time he was also getting radiation from his neck down to the pelvis from Monday to Friday. This is called Total Lymphoid Irradiation (TLI).

The ATG was actually the most painful part of the entire operation. TLI and ATG are initiated because the profound immune suppression caused by these two modalities means there is a low incidence of acute graft-versus host disease (GVHD). GVHD is a potentially serious complication of bone marrow transplantation that can affect any organ leading to severe, life-threatening damage. The transplant was actually a non-event, physically speaking. To Marty it was like a routine blood transfusion, only with a nurse coming in every fifteen minutes to check. On Friday, July 30th, Marty was taken into a chemotherapy infusion room and given blood that contained the stem cells. Because his donor was from Germany it had to be specially timed so that the stem cells were flown in just before Marty began this process. The transfusion process itself took only two hours.

Although it's technically a big event, it didn't feel like it, because compared to all the other procedures that he's had to go through, it was not visibly complicated. Major complications, if any, would come later on, not during the procedure itself.

The transplant went well, but Marty was extremely tired for the first thirty days. He still had to go in for daily blood draws and post-transplant treatments, although he was recovering so quickly that they soon pushed it to every other day. Because of his decreased immunity, he had to monitor his diet closely. The first forty days he was told to stay away from dairy products. He couldn't have fresh fruits or vegetables, except those with outer shells like bananas or oranges. Everything had to be very well cooked. Only when he got into his room at the nearby patient apartment complex, could he take off his surgical mask (provided that the doors and windows were closed). Marty was in a precarious situation. His body was vulnerable to numerous complications from the process.

Eleven days after this process was started, Marty was changed to an every other day routine for blood draws and treatments. He was ecstatic. "Can I go to a Leukemia and Lymphoma Society Support Group meeting in Modesto?" he asked his doctors. "No," they replied. They didn't want him traveling all the way to Modesto (about two hours away) so soon after the procedure. Marty agreed with them and waited until they left the room. A nurse came in. "Can I go to a support group?" he asked her. He didn't mention where it was. Thinking that it was in the hospital, she told him it was fine. Satisfied that he now had the approval from the medical staff, Marty had his reluctant mom drive him down to Modesto.

He had been going to these meetings since January 2004, as part of his mental preparation for the transplant. As he walked up to the door, he could hear voices inside. He put his ear to the door. They were talking about him.

Marty triumphantly strode into the stunned room, grinning from ear to ear, albeit through his surgical mask. He kept his distance from the group; they understood, as they were well acquainted with the bone marrow transplant process since other people in the group were also going through it. His positive attitude lifted the group. They spoke about one of his friends, Teresa, who was in the midst of preparation for a transplant that was to begin in two and a half weeks. She had a perfect bone marrow match from her sister, and was in complete remission. Her odds were as high as they could be for the situation. The group was anxious, but optimistic about her chances.

They would later find out she survived five weeks after the transplant before she died. She had developed severe graft versus host disease. This was despite having a perfect match. So the match increases your chance of not developing this complication, but doesn't guarantee safety.

Marty continued to live at the Stanford Home (a patient apartment complex) for some time. He still had to take numerous precautions, such as constant fluid hydration. He was required to drink 3 liters every day and had difficulty despite his mom being on the case. "It was really hard to get him to drink that amount. He didn't like to drink water. So I had to kind of trick him with popsicles, Jell-O, and different things. I just didn't understand why it was so hard. Finally, he got so irritated that he challenged me to do the same thing. So every day I would keep track of both of our amounts. Drinking 3 liters is a lot harder than I thought," his mom laughs.

Three months after his transplant, Marty was still staying at the Home. One night, he settled into a recliner to watch television. His mother was in the kitchen, cleaning dishes. Suddenly, Marty jumped out of his chair, screaming loudly. His mother rushed out of the kitchen to find her son clutching his head, yelling incoherently about fire and his eye. He rushed past her, into the kitchen, and flung open the freezer. He grabbed the ice cube tray and cracked it against the wall. Ice cubes flew all over the counter. He grabbed a handful and pressed them against his eyeballs. His mom watched from just a few feet away, not understanding, and powerless to help her son. "I just stood there in shock. I couldn't believe what I was seeing," she remembers.

Help came quickly and got Marty back to the hospital. As he lay in a gurney, he saw a familiar face. It was Marie's father. She was also back in the hospital. Despite the pain, Marty promised to see her. Finally he got wheeled to his room. When the doctors saw him, he had a scattered rash around his left eye. The doctors were afraid that it was graft versus host disease, appearing on his face. However, an urgent biopsy showed viral particles in the rash consistent with shingles—This was another flare of herpes zoster, but in a different area. It can precipitate in the region of the eye and cause immense pain. He was started on IV-acyclovir (an anti-viral drug). They gave him a portable drip unit, which looks like a fanny pack. It would automatically drip the anti-viral drug into him once every eight hours. Then he would go to the center every day to switch the drug pack on the portable drip unit. He had developed sores in both his eye and torso. "This was the worst pain I've felt," he says.

The pain would suddenly flare up, and pressure would well up in his eye. The pressure would be so intense he was afraid that his eyeball was about to explode. He would clutch his face as his mom cradled him on the ground, both of them unable to stop his pain. The episodes would last for only five to ten minutes, but to Marty they obviously felt a lot longer. He could never anticipate when it would occur, knowing only that it consistently happened at least twice a day. He would try forcing ice packs onto his eye, which never helped but it at least gave him a feeling that he was doing something to relieve the pain.

Amazingly, this was not the worst part of Marty's experience. It was the worst pain, but not the worst experience.

During this time, he met a fellow transplant patient, Ricky. Ricky was twenty-two years old, and had hematological problems because of a birth defect. When he was eighteen, he developed Burkitt's lymphoma (an aggressive disease). Like Marty, Ricky was full of optimism, most of it provided by youth. The two of them discussed everything they were going to do once they were out of the hospital. Marty talked so confidently about the future that sometimes Ricky thought it would be happening immediately. Once, Marty talked about how he was going to drive a bumper cart as soon as he got out. "Ricky got really excited; he thought I had carts outside the hospital ready to go," Marty laughs. Marty felt a strong bond with Ricky. They were both being put through a rigorous test of spirit that very few could empathize with.

Marty also made good on his promise and visited Marie while she was in the hospital. She had been allowed to live at home after her transplant since she lived so close. Their relationship became close. They called each other on the phone and wrote letters to one another.

What she had not revealed to him was she had already been told she was terminal, without options. The transplant had not worked for her.

Every time he visited her, she would wear a cap because the tumor had spread to her brain and scalp. Marty could tell she was having a hard time (they were injecting chemotherapy directly into her spine to relieve the pain) but he had no idea it was terminal. He called her throughout December. He wanted to see her after his full recovery. He was so optimistic about the future that the positivity was extended to all his loved ones. And with cancer, you can easily be too optimistic. One night, her mother said she couldn't come to the phone. Marie was too tired from all the treatments.

A week later he called again. Her mom picked up the phone.

"Are you ready for this, Marty?" she sobbed.

Marie had died two days earlier, on January 16th. She had made her parents promise not to tell Marty about her condition until she passed away. She had lasted five and a half months after the transplant. She was twenty-eight.

Several days later Marty found out that Ricky died on January 17th.

This began the toughest period in Marty's life, a battle with depression that brought him to his lowest point, mentally speaking. He kept asking himself why did he survive and not them? Ricky was only twenty-two, and Marie only twenty-eight. Marty was forty-five and still going strong, while these dear friends of his lost the chance to live their lives.

Marty wanted to be a martyr for cancer. But by definition, doesn't a martyr die?

He did not understand the new pain gnawing at him. He briefly considered the help of a psychologist. Finally, one night on CNN, he saw a special about military soldiers who were suffering from what is known as survivor's guilt. In wartime, within a unit or between individuals, luck plays a large role in determining who survives. Your friend took a bullet to the chest, but it could just as easily have been you. Many soldiers suffer from the guilt of knowing a good person died simply because of bad luck. The question remains in their head: Why not me? Marty has now grown to accept it, but it took several years. His depression lasted for several months. That's when he decided to volunteer at the Leukemia and Lymphoma Society. Both Marie and Ricky wanted to donate to the group.

At first, he tells me, giving back to other cancer patients was the best therapy. But there is a deeper change at work here. It is an underlying philosophy that affects him more than the passage of time or his charitable contributions and one that he understood more deeply after the birth of his children.

"I guess me being able to reproduce changed my thoughts somewhat. Although, I felt guilt initially about that as well. Again, this was an opportunity that my friends missed out on. But after a while, watching other people go through similar fights...We have to make the most of what we're given. None of us are entitled to a long, healthy life. It is up to us to make the most of what God has blessed us with. I'm content now because I've taken advantage of the extra time I've been granted. If I should die tomorrow...." He pauses. "I'm okay with that," he shrugs. He tells me this as we can hear his eleven-month-old daughter in another room playing with her dolls. He's frightfully sincere at this moment, not trying to impress either himself or me. It's not exactly fair to say that he believes God has chosen him to survive. Because the unmentioned aspect of that belief would be that some of his friends were chosen to die. But what sense does it make to feel guilt for prospering in a bleak situation? Marty's attitude might diminish the terrifying nature of his lymphoma, but even leaving out death, he still suffered greatly. Ten years of his life were spent fighting the cancer, getting his energy drained by chemotherapy and the disease, fighting the pain of the tumor pressing against his tissue and bones, and putting his friends and family though stress. So when life is gracious enough to give him some fortune, he certainly appreciates it. More importantly, there isn't a reason to feel guilty over it.

The Leukemia and Lymphoma Society holds an annual marathon called the "Rock and Roll." They also choose an honored hero to commemorate each event. Marty's story had become famous in the group and after spending so much time volunteering, he was chosen as the 2005 honored hero. Not much time had passed since his transplant, and Marty began training only ten days before the marathon. All 26.2 miles of it.

But he had been specifically chosen to represent at the marathon down in San Diego and there was no way he would let anyone down. The morning of the marathon, he received a call from his pastor wishing him luck. During that day's congregation, he was going to be the focus. Someone in the church would monitor Marty's progress on the checkpoint results the marathon published online. Marty not only had their support, but also the added responsibility to not let them down.

Marty got to work, making sure he reached each checkpoint in the allotted time. It took him over two hours to complete the last five miles of the marathon. "I felt like my calves were going to explode with each step," he remembers. The last tenth of the mile he ran to the finish line as the crowd applauded wildly.

Four days later, he met his transplant physician at Stanford. "Is it okay if I train for a marathon?" Marty asked him.

"I don't see why not," his physician replied. He asked when it was. Sunday, Marty told him. "This Sunday?" asked the incredulous doctor. "Nope. Last Sunday." A grinning Marty revealed his latest accomplishment. He showed the skeptical physician his marathon medal. It was that conversation that led to Marty being chosen by the physician to be the subject of a *Stanford Report* article that focused on the new stem cell transplant procedure. Anyone who could complete a 26-mile marathon a year after their transplant was obviously a success story.

In November 2005, Marty found himself back at Stanford for a follow-up appointment. In the parking lot, he got a call from St. Joseph's Medical Center. They wanted him to be a poster child in their ad campaign. Marty was initially nominated in October 2005 after spending time at St. Joseph's "We Can Weekend," a get together for cancer patients. His story had impressed the powers that be and they wanted him in the advertisements. They talked about his personality, his ordeal, and how he wanted to be pictured. His intensity had to be the central theme. He wanted to be "The Cancer Challenger." They settled on an image of him boxing. Like everything else, Marty took the photo shoot seriously. He trained heavily and practiced on a speed bag in his gym. By the time they were shooting in the first week of January 2006, he was in tiptop shape. The production company had rented a location for the afternoon. The boxing equipment was in an old warehouse in downtown Stockton that was converted to a boxing gym. There was no heat because the gym hadn't opened yet, and the warehouse itself was already cold. They sprayed Marty with artificial sweat (otherwise known as water) and asked him to hit the bag swinging from the right while his face had to be twisted to the left. The makeup artist repeatedly interrupted to spread foundation on his chest. She wanted to change his tan lines, fix the bags under his eyes, adjust the sweat... on and on the changes continued. They worked all day and took over 200 shots. Finally, Marty pictured the makeup artist's face on the bag and threw one punch with all his strength. That became the billboard image.

They thanked him for his time and told him the ads would be up in a couple of months. His image was finally plastered all over the county in February 2006.

"Back in 2003, I would look up at billboards as I was driving and picture myself up there," he says after seeing the initial advertisements by the hospital. "When I was nominated to be a poster child I thought this could very well happen. Just because I was nominated didn't mean I was definitely going to be chosen. There are some unbelievable stories out there." Soon people kept coming up to him to tell him they had seen him on the billboards. Some thought he really was a boxer. Two of Marty's dreams had come true. The first was that larger than life image of himself. It gave him a measure of pride to see how far he had come. The second and more important goal was feeling as though he'd given hope to others.

He met his wife, Elisa, in church during July 2005. They became good friends and he leaned on her during tough times. It's another connection with his religious faith that Marty doesn't talk about despite being a devout Christian. He admits that he's found a lot of strength through his faith. After his initial diagnosis, he attended church more frequently. Elisa, like Marty, is religious and very outgoing. The church began a cancer support group several years ago. Marty spends a lot of time there to help others by offering his insight and experience.

"When I was going through this, I personally avoided a lot of external influence because I wanted to know my true thoughts on it. How I alone felt on the situation. I never really socialized that much anyways because of my workload. People were stunned to know that I had cancer because they couldn't tell by looking at me, and this was while I was on chemotherapy," he says. Most people struck with cancer have to go through some personal introspection, but Marty had actually tackled the idea before he was diagnosed. Marty, though he never says it, was prepared for the eventuality of having the disease, simply by knowing his family history and watching his hero, his dad, suffer through it. But as for how he would respond? "I had no idea I had this strength. It was literally on the job training," he admits.

2006 was just as hectic for him. Marty would complete the marathon again, but not before attempting a 24-hour walk at the Oakdale Relay for Life in April 2006. Two weeks prior to the walk, he fell sick. Remember, it was unknown how long his immune system would remain compromised. After a few days of feeling ill, he took an antibiotic because he wanted to be in good condition for the relay.

He lost nine pounds within two days. He needed daily hydration, which allowed him to recover exactly one of the lost pounds. Naturally, he still showed up for the walk. The relay officials didn't know any of this, and when he showed up looking very slim, they mentioned how hard he must have trained. Marty just nodded. They had Red Cross staff in case of medical emergencies, so he felt he had backup in case his body gave out on him.

Five hours into his walk, a group of teenagers formed a cheering section for him in the stands. They had read about him in the local newspaper. After completion of every lap he got a roaring ovation. This went on for hours.

At the end of the day, he was only able to complete about forty-six miles and stopped at the ten and a half hour mark initially, then continued several hours later. It wasn't his goal, but for how ill he was it was "pretty good." The problem was that his ailment continued into May. By this time he was having difficulty breathing. His oncologist ordered a chest X-ray on June 2nd. Marty was still the honored member for the Stockton Leukemia and Lymphoma marathon team and was expected to represent them again at the Rock and Roll marathon. It was taking place in two days. As he was driving down to San Diego, he got a call from his oncologist. The X-ray showed that Marty had pneumonia.

The marathon would obviously place more stress on his lungs than anything else, important when you're struck with a potentially lethal lung complication. Marty felt compelled to at least do the first mile of the marathon. There were five checkpoints along the route, and a bus would pick people up who couldn't continue or didn't make the checkpoints within an allotted time. He struck a plan with his cousin who would do the first mile alongside him, and then Marty would take the bus to the end while she finished the marathon. But after the first mile, Marty felt warmed up. He decided to go another mile. Then another.

At the thirteen- mile mark, he left his cousin in the dust.

He wanted to make the 19.2 mile checkpoint so that he wouldn't have to take the bus, so he had to speed up for those last miles. A quarter of a mile away from the checkpoint, he could hear the bullhorn announcing the bus. The people on the sidelines were urging everyone to hurry up. He jogged the rest of the way just barely meeting the time. His cousin ended up taking a ride along with the other slow pokes.

Why he didn't stick with her? "She didn't move fast enough."

After those last six miles, he needed half an hour just to catch his breath as he continued walking to the end. Oddly enough, the next day he drove back home with no problems at all.

Two days after the marathon though, he began having difficulty breathing again. He had a CT scan done and then the same afternoon, his transplant doctor called him. The scan did not look good. Marty needed to get to Stanford immediately. He could barely breathe. He called Elisa to give her the news. She had been informing the rest of his friends about his condition. Meanwhile, his mom drove him down to Stanford to get checked. Marty got admitted to the hospital on Thursday morning, June 8th. The next day they performed a bronchoscopy (putting a camera in the lungs to make a diagnosis) and he was promptly started on aggressive antibiotics.

His sickness had progressed to the point where it was affecting more than his lungs. His eyes had become swollen again, and were leaking pus that acted like glue and stuck his eyelids together. So there he was, in Stanford's Intensive Care Unit, practically blind and having a hard time breathing and trying to stay still. He was coughing so violently the doctors were afraid that he might collapse a lung. Marty had only three thoughts.

The first was that he could very well die. He was in the worst shape he had ever been in. Ironically, it could be the pneumonia and not the cancer that might take him out (although it was the cancer treatments that made him susceptible to infections like pneumonia). "I thought wow, I've accomplished a lot. If I die, I die. My friends, Ricky and Marie, died at twenty-two and twenty-eight respectively. They weren't even given a chance. I've already been given two and a half years," he remembers.

His second thought was *They could very well have a dead man on the billboard.*

His third thought was the nurse, who was looking over a computer monitor, must be bored (in intensive care there is often a one to one ratio of nurses to patients). He called her over. "Do you have internet on your computer?" he asked her. She nodded.

"Can you look up the Rock and Roll Marathon?" he followed. Curious, she loaded the home page. There was a picture of Marty on the site, surprising the hell out of her.

Marty would deny doing this to impress anyone. He says he just wanted to make conversation with the nurse, because he thought her job was boring and felt sorry for her. Given the fact that he's saying this when his eyes are glued shut and his ribs and chest wall are close to breaking from coughing, I really don't believe him. Much of Marty's strength comes from the idea that he can shock people by demonstrating the strength of the human body and will. Marty wanted to be a martyr, but he ended up creating a hero. It's an image that propelled him.

Like the time he handed a ten-by-twelve picture of his billboard campaign to his transplant doctor, who showed it to his excited young son. The kid thought Marty was a professional boxer. For a while he even surfed the web trying to keep an eye on Marty's boxing career. Marty never told him the truth. It really didn't matter, because after meeting Marty, it's believable that he's a pugilist. It's the story that counts. And the idea that a man emerges from a bruising battle with cancer stronger than before is just too inspiring to pass up.

The marathon hadn't actually made his pneumonia any worse. Marty tells me that he wasn't running or exerting himself. I'll disagree on the latter. But the exercise itself didn't exacerbate the pneumonia. It exhausted him and perhaps delayed his treatment, but certainly didn't cause extra growth. It took doctors a week to identify the type of pneumonia. This illness can be fungal, bacterial, or viral. This one happened to be bacterial. He was started on an aggressive IV antibiotic regimen and gradually improved.

While he was recovering at Stanford, Marie's parents came

to visit him. "Thank you for being sick," her mother jokingly told him. This was an upsetting area to be in, to see the hospital corridors where their daughter had received treatments before she passed away. They needed to get closure though, and visiting Marty in the hospital forced them to do so. Marie's parents still keep in touch with Marty, sincerely thankful that he continues to do well.

And that was it. He left the hospital after a week. Another brush with death for Marty. Another scenario that he narrowly survived.

Stubborn—that's the first word that comes to mind in describing Marty's attitude toward change and toward succumbing to the disease. When I first listened to him, I couldn't get over how stubborn he appeared to be. For someone who is so obviously at risk for cancer, it took an awful lot of signs to get his attention. I was reminded of an old joke, where a man climbs to the roof of his house during a flood. He prays to God to come save him. Soon enough, a neighbor floats by on a raft, offering a helping hand. The man declines. "God will save me," he says. Later, a sailboat drifts by. They, too, offer a ride. The man declines again. "God will save me," he repeats. After that, a helicopter arrives at the scene. The crew tosses the man a rope and tells him to get in. He shakes his head. "God will save me," he says defiantly. Eventually the water level rises too high and he dies. At the Pearly Gates, he comes face to face with God. "Why didn't you save me?" he asks. God looks at him incredulously, "I sent you a raft, a boat, and a helicopter! What else did you want me to do?"

That's how I initially felt about Marty's story. How long would he have let that armpit tumor grow if he hadn't any knowledgeable clients advise him otherwise? How long could he have ignored that pneumonia growing in his lungs? How could someone not jump to conclusions in this day and age? But the truth is that Marty isn't delusional or stubborn, at least not in the way that I thought. He simply refused to let disease dominate him.

Perhaps the one person who has suffered tremendously watching Marty's unique approach is his mother. She didn't want her son to work so hard. During Marty's first visit to Stanford, she asked if his work exhaustion would make the cancer worse. They told her it wouldn't. But connecting the statistics and processes of science soundly with our emotions is a phenomenally hard task. It is why no matter how many times we hear that riding in an airplane is as safe as driving a car, most of us will never believe it. We think we need as much rest and enjoyment in our lives as possible to face a terminal illness. Marty went into battle, knowing that his lungs and heart were fine, and they would let him continue life as normal. "My mind is willing, even if the body will not respond," he says.

After the doctors had approved Marty's work schedule, his mom knew she wouldn't be able to change his mind. "He always says that he feels better when he pushes himself and gets things done," she says.

That's what it boils down to. It is the reason Marty's story is so important. Society has determined that we have to be positive when dealing with a terminal disease. Why? Let's say there is compelling data that shows optimistic people tend to live longer with a terminal disease than the pessimistic. Who cares?

Marty's ferocity was the right attitude for him because that's what makes him comfortable. Maybe just as it's right to be positive, it's also okay to wallow in misery if that's who you are naturally. It's hard being optimistic when you're not. It's hard to adopt a positive attitude that you don't believe in. I've seen patients reprimanded by friends and family for not being positive enough. Imagine being blamed for your poor condition because others think your attitude isn't right. It is tragic. People have to be who they are instead of being shackled into this existential conformity. Marty's attitude might be too positive for some people, but it's not too positive for him. And in the end that is what matters: embracing your persona during the battle for your life.

It's why getting married wasn't just a priority, but an obsession for Marty during his remission. He wanted a wife and a family. He was told by his physicians that in all likelihood he would never have kids. Intense chemotherapy and radiation often leads to infertility. You go through cancer, and despite all the support from your parents and siblings, you can still feel lonely. He wanted to find someone special.

Thinking about it, he decided he already had. "I decided why not marry my best friend? Isn't that what it is supposed to be instead of this fantasy soul mate most people envision?" he chuckles. In December 2006, he married Elisa. The following year his wife delivered their first child, Joshua. Fourteen months later she gave birth to a daughter, Haley. As always, Marty worked hard at his goals.

Marty spends a lot of time talking to cancer support groups and offering advice on an individual level. I ask him if people get upset with him. Do his views rattle people already on the edge? He pauses to consider this. It's unsettling to think that your own attitude, as natural and innocent as it may be, can upset other people so much.

If we were to sum up his philosophy, we could describe it as "the opportunity to fight cancer was a privilege and ultimately made my life better." It's not exactly an attitude most share. But after talking to him, it begins to make sense. Marty has considered the impact of his words. He has to. He tests people initially to see how strong they are emotionally. He doesn't want to scare people away, and even in the brief profiles written about him in local newspapers and support group bulletins, he shies away from saying what he really feels. "I look at it one way, that the cancer is in you for one reason and one reason only: to kill you, to blow you off the face of this earth…Most people don't want to hear that," he admits. No kidding. But it's the truth. And Marty has found that people in general are becoming stronger when it comes to dealing with cancer. People know they are not alone anymore. It's becoming easier to counsel patients. Although sometimes, you still have to walk on eggshells around them. He tries to convince them that their life could be so much worse.

Things could be so much worse? Again, it's a difficult concept to grasp, though it's a common phrase. And if you've just been given a biological death sentence, you really don't want to hear people tell you that. But if you consider his timeline, for a while, every time Marty may have thought things couldn't get worse, they would. His lowest point came after his treatment via stem cell transplant, when he witnessed close friends dying from the same process. His tailspin into depression was the only time that he was mentally beaten. So Marty has seen an ugly side of life turn even uglier. He'll tell people about the shingles in the eye, the most physically painful episodes he's had, to make them feel glad they don't have it.

He finds himself giving advice to people who don't have cancer, all the time. Someone will come up to him and ask "How do you take it on?" As if there's some profound epiphany that he can divulge. Marty simply shrugs. "It wasn't an option."

He's chosen to be a "hero of hope" for the American Cancer Society, so that he can do public speaking engagements. He's finally coped well with his survivor's guilt, in part because he's found other people who have survived the stem cell transplant, like his friend Richard, whom he met through the Leukemia & Lymphoma Society Support Group. Richard can't be in the sun much and still has to wear gloves on his hands for protection, but at least he is alive. There is such a wide variety of luck, or misfortune, not only in the diagnosis of cancer but also its treatment. Marty also still takes precautions, even though he has handled the procedure well. It's vital for him to wear sunscreen when outside because of the transplant and the dangers that ultraviolet light poses to him.

"Nowadays, every year new treatments are made available," he says excitedly. Every year is more hope and more understanding of this deadly disease. But he asked himself what would it be like if there weren't new treatments? What if there were no support groups? If he faced the issue of his mortality head on, at the young age of thirty-eight, he knew that he could live his life comfortably.

That's the secret to Marty's happiness or at the very least, his satisfaction. He never pretended that he didn't have cancer. He also didn't pretend that it couldn't kill him at any time. Have you heard the phrase "Live every day as if it's your last"? That's advice commonly given to people with terminal illnesses or to the people hearing their story. Marty ignored that. He didn't make a bucket list. He didn't take a trip to Vegas or the Caribbean and blow through his life savings. He continued to work. He basically stayed the same. Marty simply accepted the fact that he had cancer. Lymphoma was an oppressor that he couldn't run or hide from. So he took it head on. He needed an army to fight the battle. His army was the medical system. He put his full faith in them, and was confident to let them handle the worrying.

"I've had one client of mine say to me that I was in denial until I think she finally understood where I was coming from and she ended up helping me get involved with the church. There is hope out there. I have to be careful on how I say it. People said I might have gone a little cocky," he tells me. He's neither cocky or in denial though. To be "the cancer challenger," he couldn't lose. If he had died, all his money would have gone to his relatives to make their lives better. He primed his business while he was on chemotherapy and left it in a strong condition for his nephew when he could no longer continue. Being a martyr for cancer didn't mean that Marty would give up his life because of cancer; it meant that he would fight for his values. Fights aren't meant to be won with one desperate swing; they're struggles of endurance, clear-headed thinking, and heart. Marty knows all about that. He deserves to be on billboards, a bigger than life hero. He's every bit the martyr he wanted to be.

The Snowball

EVEN FATAL DISEASES have deceptively benign beginnings. A disease as serious as malaria starts with a mosquito bite. That's all it takes, one little peck of the skin by an insect that you're not likely to notice in the night. Similarly, a cancer can start off with the corruption of one cell. Think about that—something that you need a microscope to see could eventually lead to your death. People have survived stabbings, multiple bullet wounds, natural disasters, and explosions…yet the replication cycle of a cell may be beyond their means to endure. How does this happen? What is it about the nature of disease that causes severe deterioration of the body?

Enter the snowball effect. Disease, and just as important, our treatments, have direct and indirect effects. You fix one leak to find that another has been created. There is a perverse sense of risk and benefit with each move that can be made. And like a snowball rolling down a hill, the medical problems created by one little cell accumulate over time until finally there is too much momentum to stop.

In many ways, medicine is a gambling game. It only seems as though doctors have all the information. They don't. In fact, the very practice of medicine is actually detective work where evidence is gathered, usually based on a physician's hunch, and then directed into a solution. It's part lottery, part science. You can end up doing too much or maybe too little. It is sometimes hard to know which is which.

Part of this issue comes from two major obstacles. The first is risk, which comes with even the most minor of procedures or medications. Take a biopsy, for example. Stick a thin needle in to suck out a bit of tissue – this doesn't seem too dangerous. But a blood vessel could be nicked by the needle and lead to bleeding. The site of the biopsy could become infected. These would be rare complications. The point is not to be scared by the potential for rare catastrophes, but more to illustrate that there is no free lunch in medicine. The balance of pros and cons with every move is always being weighed.

The other limit is the actual ability of the physician to help patients. Despite the leaps in technology that have catapulted medicine forward, physicians are still frustrated by a myriad of problems. The most important is the inability to *cure* many diseases such as diabetes, arthritis, etc. When the aim is to treat and not cure, then the doctor is attempting to sustain life as long as possible without causing too many side effects.

That brings us to Vanessa. You see, her diagnosis of colon cancer seemed textbook. To her physicians, it felt like it should have been a simple case. Maybe it was. But just because it is simple does not mean you are in control. The truth is that because there is still so much mystery in medicine, conservative approaches toward healing the body are generally a smart way to approach most illnesses and wounds. In her story we are going to examine why average life expectancies are actually averages and not specific to a person, and why prognosis and expected side effects don't tell the whole story. What we have are options and possibilities, and while the former is limited the latter is infinite.

I have to apologize in advance about the amount of medical terminology, but we go in depth in this story to show how things can escalate despite the best intentions.

Most importantly we'll see how a microscopic clump of cells can overwhelm a person.

Vanessa, a pleasant, middle-aged woman with a shock of white hair was retired from a long stint in the trucking industry (I don't know why, but almost every patient is referred to as either pleasant or delightful by the doctor in their medical charts. I've also seen "very delightful" which I think means you're sleeping with the physician). Born in Oakland, CA in 1948, she was raised in San Leandro, part of the Northern California Bay Area. Her father was an electrician and her mother was a waitress. Both died by the age of fifty-three, from non-cancer related causes. She had two younger sisters; neither one had any issues with cancer. In fact, at the time of her diagnosis, there was no history of cancer within her family.

After she graduated from college, the best job she could find was data input on electronic keycards for the fledgling computer industry. During her brief time in that field, a friend told her that jobs in the trucking business were paying $2.10 an hour. She jumped at the opportunity and was soon hired by Pacific Inter-Mountain Express. She was there for a while, as she climbed the corporate ladder first to an office management position and then to branch manager. Frustrated with the daily commute, she quit and found a new job at a closer company, Yellow Freight trucking. Initially she was in a clerical position as part of the Teamsters union. After ten years on the job, she was promoted to the position of dispatch supervisor. Though this was a promotion, it also moved her out of the union, and with that departure she lost some of the union's benefits such as her healthcare insurance.

Several years into this new position, during April 1993, at the age of forty-five, she was startled to notice blood in her stools. She felt fine otherwise, so she ignored it for a while. "Like most silly people, I went through an initial period of self-diagnosis," she says. It isn't an unreasonable reaction, especially considering how common rectal ailments like hemorrhoids are.

After two months of bloody stools, though, Vanessa finally decided that she ought to get it checked out. She booked an appointment with her family doctor. Although something as simple as hemorrhoids might be the most common reason for this issue, physicians actually have to be concerned about a wide variety of problems. Of utmost importance is finding the source of bleeding. It is easy to assume that it is coming from the rectal area, but in fact blood could be from anywhere along the gastrointestinal (GI) tract. This tract begins in the mouth and ends in the anus. Think of it as an open tunnel going throughout your body in which food is digested and nutrients absorbed. Potential sources could be anything from peptic ulcer disease to colon cancer to hemorrhoids. Any bleeding in the gastrointestinal tract is usually classified between upper and lower, with the medical benchmark between the two being a point in the small intestine. Usually, if the bleeding comes from the upper GI tract, for example stomach ulcers, then the stools are black in color. If the bleeding is coming from what is considered the lower GI tract, then you can see bright, fresh red blood in the stool.

Vanessa had been observing red blood when she went to

the bathroom. Though it could be hemorrhoids, a more serious source of bleeding had to be ruled out.

Beyond that, the risk of colon cancer increases greatly around the age of fifty. Although Vanessa hadn't reached fifty, she was nearing that territory. This required a more thorough work-up.

With this in mind, her doctor immediately referred her to a gastroenterologist for a colonoscopy.

Colonoscopies are procedures where a camera is inserted through the anus to go up into the colon. It's done under mild anesthesia as an outpatient procedure. Before the procedure, a sedative is injected. It lasts for a short time, but people can sometimes shrug off the anesthesia and remain awake through the colonoscopy. Vanessa resisted the anesthesia immediately, and was awake throughout the entire process. Slightly dazed, she watched the small television monitor to her side as the doctor guided the camera through her intestine.

"It looked like a pink tunnel, segmented by rings. All of a sudden you see this ugly, clump of crap. Yellow and red…" as Vanessa describes it. It was only 4 cm (about one and half inches) in size but on the monitor it looked gigantic. And hearing Vanessa explain, it might as well have been 4 meters wide. "That's causing your bleeding," the doctor told her.

In the recovery room, Vanessa went over what happened with her husband, Andrew. He's a former navy officer who works for Pac Bell. The gastroenterologist entered the room, and told them he was almost certain that the ugly mass was a cancer. It was an educated guess (only a biopsy and examination under a microscope can definitely confirm a malignancy), but the word "cancer" drops like a bombshell in the room. Unless it was negated by biopsy results, in Vanessa's mind she had cancer.

"It is just unbelievable. I couldn't believe it was happening to me," she sobs as she reminisces about an event that happened nearly two decades ago. "The thing was, I wanted it out, right [then]. It's like you just picture—there is this connotation of cancer and you picture it spreading everywhere. I found out later that it was a slow-growing cancer and I probably had it for years. They couldn't get me in for at least two weeks for the surgery. But after I found I had cancer, they couldn't do the surgery fast enough as far as I was concerned.

"I did not know anybody that had cancer. And everything you heard about cancer was that it was very painful. That chemotherapy was horrible. That you threw up all the time. There is old wives' tale that surgery can spread the cancer. The whole process was very terrifying. You automatically think you are going to die, and you think you are going to die soon. You don't think you are going to be a survivor because you don't know anyone that survived. It was a shock to begin with because when I went in for the colonoscopy I wasn't thinking about cancer. I thought I had colitis. It just took my breath away to think I had cancer."

Several days later, the biopsy sample taken during colonoscopy confirmed her fears. While most people could only imagine what their cancer looked like, Vanessa had actually seen it on the television monitor. Did this exacerbate her anxiety? In her mind, she pictured the ugly mass moving, spreading throughout her body. As with most other people, Vanessa assumed that the progression to the sickly, emaciated life would happen with the same speed that she had received this diagnosis. Neither Vanessa nor her husband understood what was going on. Even more difficult would be breaking the news to their daughter, a senior in high school, who was waiting at home. But Vanessa didn't think about that.

"Initially, it's about you," she says. "After a while, it becomes about them." "Them" being family and friends. But at the time, the cancer's effects on her and her alone were first and foremost in her mind. It's not that it eventually left her thoughts; it never would, but over time it became a secondary focus. It was a feeling replicated in her family. The focus was Vanessa. Her husband and daughter cared only about what would happen to her, not what would happen to them once she was gone.

When Vanessa says this, she's not mincing words. She can describe in detail the colonoscopy and how the doctor broke the news to her. She remembers her immediate reaction. You would expect her to remember the response of her loved ones as well. But ask her to remember what her husband's reaction was like or even how the two of them broke the news to their daughter, and she can't describe it. It's doubtful she could have described it the day after the colonoscopy. She simply didn't pay attention to it. There's an emotional fog during this time period, hiding everyone's story but hers.

Let's face it; while most of us have fears of dying and think about it once in a while, it is an entirely different mental process when there is weight behind those thoughts. "You can just be driving down the road, and your mind is wandering and all of sudden you are thinking, how long am I going to live?" she says. Being faced with a realistic possibility of death in the near future is not just scary, it is overwhelming. This mindset would dictate many of her decisions.

What Vanessa didn't know was that her cancer was growing slowly…so slowly that she could have waited months before getting surgery without any deleterious effect to her long-term survival. Even if she'd had that knowledge, though, it's doubtful that Vanessa would have settled for anything less than the earliest possible date for her procedure. That initial fear was too compelling.

Her surgery had been scheduled two weeks after the colonoscopy. It was also the same time that her daughter, a senior golfer who was on the varsity team at her high school, had been invited to the World Junior tournament held annually in San Diego. It was the same weekend as Vanessa's surgery. It seems obvious that Vanessa's daughter would skip it. But when you think about it, once a person's life expectancy is dramatically shortened, those golf tournaments for your children are the kind of events you don't want to miss.

So how would surgery help Vanessa? In addition to removing the primary tumor and surrounding tissues it would also provide information on how far it had spread. This would allow her physicians to stage the disease.

Surgery in these cases is done with a curative intent. The term cure means that your life expectancy is the same as somebody who does not have the cancer. Some people are cured with surgery alone. For Stage I colon cancer the cure rate is 95%, for Stage II it is 80%, and Stage III it is about 50%.

During her surgery, nineteen lymph nodes in the pelvic region were removed and tested for cancer. One was positive. Although the other eighteen were free of cancer, that one lymph node involvement meant she had Stage III disease. Stage III means that the chance of the cancer returning in the next five years is usually more than 50%. This meant that there was a 50% chance that there were cancer cells somewhere else in the body that were too small to be detected by any scans or blood tests. These cancer cells would continue to divide and over a period of time form tumors. Vanessa would require treatment to kill these cancer cells that were undetectable by technology. That would require chemotherapy, injected intravenously, to course throughout the body and hopefully kill residual cancer cells. Such treatment (called adjuvant chemotherapy—treatment given immediately after surgery) decreases the chances of the cancer coming back by about half. Vanessa needed chemotherapy as a means of decreasing the risk of recurrence for a cancer that may or may not have existed.

A CEA (carcino-embryonic antigen) blood test level pre- and post-surgery was normal, and would also be normal at the completion of her chemotherapy. A CEA test measures the amount of a protein that appears in the blood of some people who have certain kinds of cancers. It is commonly used to follow colon cancer, although its level can also go up in other cancers, such as those of the breast, ovary, lung, and pancreas. So it is not specific for any particular malignancy. There are also non-cancerous conditions that can lead to a high CEA level, including cigarette smoking, liver cirrhosis, inflammatory bowel disease, chronic lung disease, and pancreatitis. In fact, three percent of the healthy population will have a high CEA level. Therefore it is not always a reliable test for cancer and not used to diagnosis the initial disease or estimate stage. Its main use is to help diagnose colon cancer recurrence, which you do by comparing it to the baseline. If a CEA level gradually goes up, it may suggest very early recurrence, and would prompt scans or other tests to look for evidence of a new growth.

Vanessa's options for follow-up treatment were limited compared to today. She was set to receive chemotherapy for one year with the drug 5-Fluouracil (5 Fu). That was the only drug available at that time; there was nothing else for colon cancer. At the end of the year the treatment would be complete, and the waiting would begin. If the cancer came back, it would normally do so within five years. If it did, then she had no realistic options for a cure. After five years, the statistical chances of the cancer coming back were low, though not zero (it was less than 5%). There were no other alternatives or timelines to consider. [1]

She spent one hour every week in the chemotherapy unit. She would sit by herself and ponder the randomness of life and why this was happening to her.

Her chemotherapy clinic was not as active as it is today. "Back when I first had to do chemo there were only three recliner chairs [in the clinic]. You never saw anyone but medical personnel. You didn't see other patients," she remembers. This was both a blessing and a curse. On one hand, Vanessa didn't want to know anything else about the disease. She was trying her hardest to pretend she didn't have it. To not see other people suffering from cancer made it easier for her to ignore her own ailment. On the other hand, cancer is a lonely disease. Other people can't understand what you're going through, and everyone treats you differently. Morbid as it sounds, it can be helpful to know that other people have gone through similar battles.

During that year of treatment, Vanessa had several goals.

---

1 You might be wondering why it's one year. The timeline actually is not specific to Vanessa. An initial study that showed that giving chemotherapy after surgery to patients with Stage III colon cancer showed a survival advantage of 40%. The chemotherapy was given for one year. The one-year period was chosen empirically by the physicians who crafted the study. Subsequent studies have shown that similar chemotherapy given for six months as compared to one year is equally effective. Nowadays, chemotherapy after surgery in colon cancer is given only for six months. The truth is that there is actually no marker to see how she is responding to treatment. Protocols are established through research. Originally, the only treatment was surgical removal of the tumor, but as we now know, that removes only the cancer cells that the doctors can see. This would create a 50% chance of survival without recurrence after five years in Stage III disease. Then chemotherapy entered the scene, and improved the chances to approximately 75%, but only if applied to all patients. So even those who might not need chemotherapy would sometimes get it. Addition of chemotherapy after Stage III disease improves your odds of survival by about 40%.

Among them was to maintain a sense of normalcy. By that, I mean maintaining the life she had before cancer. Some people, such as Marty, consider their fight with cancer to have positively changed aspects of their life. But most others, like Vanessa, would do anything to return to that world that existed before cancer. So the next best thing is to imagine a life without cancer. And in that life, nothing changes. That's why "normalcy" was so important to her. One of the ways she maintained it was through her job.

Midway through that year of chemotherapy, Vanessa was in her fourth year as a manager with Yellow Freight. Her job was to organize delivery loads for trucks on the weekends. When she was diagnosed with cancer, she informed upper management that she was going to be off for roughly two months following her major surgery and that she would return to work afterwards. She was able to follow that timeline, but the standard schedule for that position was 50+ hours a week. Still recuperating from surgery and being initiated into the world of chemo, Vanessa didn't have it in her to keep that workload. She was able to strike a deal to work 40 hours a week. This arrangement lasted from September 1993 to April 1994, and during that time span she only missed three days of work.

During April, still on chemotherapy, she was sent to Kansas City to fulfill one of the other parts of her job, which was reallocation of people injured while working and who were placed on worker's comp. Vanessa supervised a process to figure out work for these non-union employees, which they could perform with their injury. During the middle of this session, word leaked out that the Teamsters had gone on strike. Vanessa wasn't part of the union, but without their cooperation, no other work could go on. When she returned home, she and the other employees were told that they could either take a vacation or be let go. Vanessa chose the former.

During her "vacation," Vanessa received a call that she had been let go anyway. She didn't fret about it, figuring once the strike was over everyone would be recalled back to work. "At the time, it was very important to retain normalcy in my life. I wanted things to go back to the way they were. Which wasn't going to happen, but it was important to have as much normal as I could," Vanessa says.

Vanessa went on disability, and waited to hear back. She would talk to coworkers and hear about people slowly being recalled back to the company. Only her turn never came. The more time that passed without her being recalled, the more she began to suspect that she had been laid off permanently. The biggest clue came when she got word that the company had brought back a person in her position who had been with the business for only six months in that department (remember, she had been there for three years). Finally, she got a call from HR in the corporate office in Tracy, a nearby city, saying she might be hearing from some of the other managers in the area for possible positions.

"Here they were, recalling people with less time, supervisors that I know did not get as good reviews as I did, so I knew what was going on," she bristles.

She was never given an excuse. Finally, she was offered a position to be a dock supervisor at night. The shift required her to be at the loading stations from about 4 in the afternoon till the next morning. Between chemotherapy treatments and looking after her daughter, she obviously couldn't manage that. I'll let you piece together what the company was doing, and Vanessa's subsequent lawsuit and settlement certainly removed any mystery after that.

"I'm still very irritated about that," she says somberly. She should be. Her hard work and loyalty to the company were washed down the drain at the first convenient opportunity. You get cancer and you expect at least that everyone will treat you with courtesy and respect. Vanessa had found that was not the case.

She was relegated to her home for the full duration of treatment. The stress was alleviated by the fact that her husband's job provided healthcare benefits for their family, and she had the opportunity to spend more time with her daughter, who was a senior in high school, and would be off to college in a year. Vanessa was afraid that she might not survive to see her daughter attend Oregon State.

But in fact, she managed to do better than any of her wildest expectations. She breezed through the chemotherapy, only rarely feeling the common side effects such as nausea and fatigue. A year went by during which she had good health.

After that one year of chemotherapy, the treatment was stopped. Vanessa continued her quest for the grail of normalcy once again. And lady luck finally looked her way. She got a call in September from an acquaintance in the trucking industry, working for a company in Manteca (roughly 20 minutes driving distance from Stockton). He offered her a temporary job in management, and when that stint was over she was recommended for a position in an Oakland office for clerical work. Vanessa was back with the Teamsters.

She had found her normalcy, turning back the clock to a time when she didn't have the disease. The only caveat was that she was required to see her oncologist every six months for at least five years. Why only five years? Statistically, after five years of being in remission, the chances of having a recurrence are very low, much lower than 5%. After those five years, if she was still negative for the disease, she no longer had to see the oncologist. Theoretically, there was almost no chance of the colon cancer recurring.

Vanessa remained anxious about her condition. Statistics didn't completely assure her. But five years went by without any sign of the cancer. Her health had no hiccups of any kind. Her oncologist had told her she no longer had to see him. She had a clean bill of health. So when she asked her primary care physician to keep running the CEA test during an annual checkup, he was somewhat surprised. Even doing a CEA test after completion of chemotherapy is controversial, as it is unclear whether doing this test really saves any lives. The CEA test isn't even normally run in most cancer cases, and here Vanessa was asking her primary care physician to run it for her. Not only that— she had passed the safe stage according to all standard practices. But she had grown accustomed to using the CEA as a baseline way of gauging her health, as her own bodily intuition had failed long ago to notify her of the cancer's presence.

So from 1998 to 2001, she asked her primary care physician to check her CEA levels on a yearly basis. Post-chemotherapy it was less than 1.0. In mid-2000, her CEA was 1.6. That's a slight increase but still within normal range.

In September 2001, it rose to 6.2.

A normal level for CEA is less than 5. An alarmed Vanessa practically ran to her oncologist, so tests could be run to look for visible evidence of recurrence. Every possible test or scan that could be used to confirm it was utilized. "We would run a blood test and other things every three months —and the PET scan had just come out. None of the facilities had the machinery, and it was in these mobile truck trailers," she remembers (the only PET scanner in town came in a truck one day a week to save on cost).

Every test came back negative. Except for the gradually increasing CEA level, there was no visible indication that Vanessa's cancer had returned. We've already discussed the potential fallacies of CEA levels. To her doctors it was unclear whether this really signified the early return of her cancer. The slowly rising CEA level could also have been related to a non-cancerous condition. It was possible that it was just inflammation in the body. Perhaps it was a wild goose chase that was destroying poor Vanessa's peace of mind. With no real way of knowing, her doctors advised her to wait a couple of months and see if anything changed.

On March 15th 2003, she returned for a check-up and had another CEA test run. It had risen to 22.

I've reproduced the progression of her CEA levels below:

September 1999—-0.4
September 2000—-1.6
September 2001—-6.2
April 2002—-6.5
June 2002—-6.9
October 2002—-12.1
March 2003—-22

Although nothing else had changed and this still could be a false positive, Vanessa underwent testing again. CT scans of her abdomen and pelvis were normal. So was a repeat PET scan. She had another colonoscopy performed in April 2003. That was also normal.

"You name it and they tried it," she laughs.

You need to understand that there are limits, major ones in fact, in the tools available in medicine. Most people do not understand that you can have a cancerous tumor growing in the body and yet feel absolutely normal and healthy. Your blood tests and scans can be normal in the beginning stages of most cancers. For most tumors we do not have good means of detecting them early on. For example, in order for X-rays and scans (CT, MRI, and PET) to spot a tumor, it needs to be of a certain size. It takes one billion cancer cells to create a tumor about 1 cm in size. So if you have a 100 million cancer cells in one spot, you can do all the scans in the world and it will still not show anything. Even when it is beyond one centimeter in size, a fair amount of disease can still be missed on the scan. Even with bulky disease, the scans usually underestimate the amount of disease present in the body. So a rising CEA level could be produced by cancer cells incapable of being visualized by our present imaging technology. Unfortunately, most people think tests can pick up any evidence of cancer or illnesses in general. A normal scan doesn't mean absence of disease; it means the absence of visible disease.

By 2003, Vanessa had become anxious, frustrated, and upset.

She was eventually sent to USCF (University of California San Francisco) for another opinion. A CT scan of the chest was done at UCSF which showed a nodule, 2cm in size, in the right lung (a scan done a few months ago had not shown it). A CT guided needle biopsy was performed. It showed cells consistent with a metastatic colon cancer that had spread to the lung.

Vanessa had bucked the five-year rule. Now it was back to the fight. Since the lung nodule was the only visible site of disease, the plan was to remove it surgically. Physicians ran Vanessa through a battery of tests to gauge things like lung capacity and heart function to make sure she could survive the procedure.

In December 2003, they removed a portion of the middle lobe of her right lung (you have two lungs, right and left. Each is divided into parts called lobes. The right lung has three lobes—upper, middle, and lower—while the left lung has only an upper and lower lobe).

In the final part of the procedure, the surgeon had to make an incision on the right side of her torso and insert drainage tubes so the fluid in the cavity could be removed (this fluid comes from multiple sources like the cancer, lungs, blood vessels, etc.). These tubes remain in place until they no longer drain fluid. They can be quite painful.

"The nerve centers, you have a lot more apparently in the sides, so…for a few days after, while I was still in the hospital, was extremely painful. I had an epidural pain blocker. But sometime in the first day after the surgery it came out so the pain was no longer blocked. I was in a university hospital, they have teams, and there was virtually nothing they could do since it was in the middle of the night. The pain took my breath away, it was so bad. I would have done anything for them to get the tube out."

It was night and Andrew had left the room to return to his hotel and sleep. The pain management physicians wouldn't return till morning. There was nothing for Vanessa to do but grit and bear the pain through that long night with only the TV for company. The next morning they removed the drainage tubes from her back and the pain subsided.

Deciding to do surgery was the easy part. It was the follow-up treatment that was unclear. The only visible disease was the solitary spot in the right lung. There was a possibility that surgery was the only treatment required. Her oncologist recommended a baseline CEA post-surgery and then to follow it every three to four months to see if the CEA levels would gradually disappear (it takes between three to four months for the body to stop producing CEA if it has become relatively cancer-free).

Vanessa waited. In March 2004, she went back for another CEA level.

The CEA had actually gone up. It was now 28.

It was time to search for the cancer again.

Vanessa underwent a PET scan. It showed major new changes in her abdomen, suggestive of cancer in multiple lymph nodes in her belly. This was turning out to be an unusually complicated scenario. Vanessa went back to University of California, San Francisco Medical Center for further recommendations.

There are multiple reasons to send a patient to a university center. It doesn't necessarily mean the patient's physician doesn't know how to handle the case. With an unusual disease pattern, there is the potential for more complications than normal. Universities are often sent these types of complex cases as they have more experience with them. Beyond that, the patient gets the reassurance that they are receiving another good opinion from a reliable institution.

The surgical oncologist at UCSF saw Vanessa and then told her that he wanted his own team to run another CT scan. Unfortunately, Vanessa had switched to a different HMO recently. In this HMO's policy, the scans would be covered only if they were run locally in town with facilities they had a contract with. The HMO felt that a CT scan done locally should be as good as it would be in any university center. The university facilities were not part of the HMO contract. So, although the university physicians had a contract with the HMO, the radiology facility in the university was not part of the deal. Despite the power and prestige of the UCSF cancer center, their physicians didn't have enough power to compel her insurance company.

Finally, after much haggling, a compromise was reached where the scans would be run locally but with imaging cuts recommended by the USCF oncological surgeon. "Cuts" refers to the heights of the body where the scan is taking place. CT scans basically look at a thin image of the body at a certain height, as if you had sliced a person in half and looked from the top of the body. Slices are done at different depth intervals— for example 0.5 cm or 1 cm.

Vanessa went in for the scan, and waited for word that her local scanning facility had sent the images to the university. Every day, she called the university to check if they had received the scans. For two weeks the answer was no. Finally, she went over to the center where they performed the CT. The images were lying in a drawer on the front desk. She yanked them from the secretary's hand and sent it to UCSF herself through overnight mail.

"It was very frustrating; nobody seemed to care," she remembers.

Vanessa anxiously waited until the next morning. The scans weren't going to show anything new for her, but the results could help determine further treatment options. She was desperate to know the next step.

The next day, she dialed the UCSF office. The nurse who answered her call checked the records and confirmed the office had received the images.

"Well, what did the doctor think?" Vanessa asked.

"He said it's inoperable. You need to go on chemotherapy." That would be the extent of their conversation.

This anti-climactic interaction disturbed Vanessa greatly. "I was just never happy. I always felt that they didn't look at it. Because they didn't have their own radiologists to read it and it was just too quick, you know? The doctor didn't talk to me, it was one of the nurses," she tells me. She thought perhaps the surgeon's frustration in dealing with the insurance issues had colored his opinion of her case.

Now, in reality, there is next to no chance the doctor's exasperation with the HMO situation affected his medical decision (if frustration with insurance caused spiteful medical decisions, no one would receive proper care). Whether or not his team conducted the scans, the advice offered would be the same. In fact, it was the same recommendation offered by Vanessa's local oncologist.

Yet Vanessa's frustrations with this situation may have colored her interpretation of the course of her cancer. These are frustrations that many other patients share. Many have a paranoid mindset. Vanessa's cancer, as we will see, continued to recur. And at the end of a long fight, if you are losing, you start to go over the small turns that you think could have affected the outcome. Her unease at this doctor's method of communication, the small gut instinct that something was not right there, sticks with her. It shapes and colors her experience, a fact that is magnified as her depiction of this time period is different than what is present on her medical records. Her own oncologist felt the decision to give chemotherapy was the right choice. He did not truly feel that Vanessa was a surgical candidate at that point in time.

"I pursued that abdominal surgery. You know when they tell you something is inoperable it is like giving up. To me it was like they were giving up on me, or there was nothing they could do.

That maybe wasn't totally true, because you still get chemo, but it still felt if you could take it out, then you had a better chance," Vanessa laments.

The argument the UCSF physician made, and one that Vanessa's local oncologist agreed with, was that it would not be in her best interest to operate and "debulk" the disease. Surgical debulking is exactly what it sounds like: a surgeon going in and removing cancerous tissue surgically. The benefit of debulking as opposed to chemotherapy is that it may take a long time for the disease to grow back for someone like Vanessa who is known to have a slow-growing cancer. The disadvantage of this major surgery is that you can have major, life-threatening complications including infection, bleeding, etc.

And remember, scans often underestimate the amount of disease. When surgeons go inside the body, they can find more disease than anticipated. If there is too much cancer present, they close the person back up because the procedure will be an ineffective measure. This doesn't change the fact that the patient has undergone surgery, in this case with no meaningful benefit, and now has to recuperate from the process of being put under anesthesia and cut open. This recuperation period can delay further treatment.

The other option in Vanessa's case was to receive chemotherapy and if the disease shrank well, then reconsider surgery with less volume of disease. This is termed chemical debulking. It was the option her medical practitioners advised.

It was 2005, twelve years after she first had chemotherapy and Vanessa was set to play the game once again. It is extremely unusual to have such a long disease-free interval in patients with colon cancer.

In those twelve years, new chemotherapy drugs had become available. Vanessa was started on a combination of chemotherapy drugs, with the acronym FOLFIRI (5-fluorouracil, Irinotecan, and Leucovorin calcium). She had used only 5-fluoruracil in 1993 and responded well. She would see dramatic improvement again with the new combination.

But if a person responds so well to treatment, why does the cancer keep returning?

Chemotherapy is capable of killing only a certain percentage of cancer cells each time it is given. Remember, chemo drugs are toxic not only to cancer cells, but also to normal cells. There is only a certain amount that you can administer at one time into a person's body. On the other hand, the number of cancer cells can be huge. This presents a problem because the limited amount of chemo you can inject guarantees you won't kill all the cancer cells. Patients need time to recuperate from each drug infusion. During this period, the cancer continues to do what it did before and will always do: replicate. And with such a large number of cells, even if you kill 50%, it doesn't take too long for the cells to replicate back to their previous number and grow even more numerous. This is why the cycles of chemotherapy have to be given persistently.

Vanessa was stunned by the turn of events. She had been so close to "victory," and yet she was forced relive her original nightmare.

"There were times in between treatments where I couldn't stand to look at an IV pole. I can remember seeing pictures where they were advertising medications and it just turned my stomach. I think I was in my living room reading some magazines and seeing somebody in a hospital bed with an IV pole… it just made me sick."

She was amazed by the changes to the medical system that had manifested in the new decade. In 1993, she had been an outlier. In the 2000s, she was another drop in the bucket of malignancy increasingly recognized as a common ailment. "It blew me away when I went to chemotherapy [twelve] years later to walk in and see thirty chairs all full of people getting chemotherapy. Because they didn't have that office back then. I couldn't believe that it had gotten so bad that there was all these people, but then you start to realize it's not that there are more people, but that people are living longer and there is more you can do about them. It's sad and then it's not. A lot of these people go on to live a long life afterwards."

After six months of Vanessa responding well to the treatment, a scan showed dramatic shrinkage of disease. In fact there was barely anything visible on the PET scan. Vanessa's oncologist began to entertain the idea of surgical debulking once again. He consulted an oncological surgeon. They agreed the benefit, if it worked out, would be consolidation of Vanessa's chemotherapeutic gains. The disease had already shrunk dramatically, and they knew by its history that it was a slow-growing disease. If they could surgically remove the remaining cancerous tissue that had not responded to the chemotherapy, theoretically it could give Vanessa even more time before its resurgence. The expectation of treatment was not to cure the disease, but to give Vanessa a long disease-free interval where she would be symptom-free, independent of treatment, and could live a normal life.

Performing the surgery would also give them an opportunity to reconfirm the presence and type of cancer. This seems odd, since she had been told so many times she had metastatic colon cancer. So why would they need to reconfirm it?

The fact of the matter is that Vanessa's case, with its pattern of spread and the long disease-free interval, was highly unusual. There are so many things that can go wrong in the human body, and many of these ailments overlap in their symptoms. This seemed like a reasonable way to confirm everything, by getting more tissue and examining it under the microscope, with the added benefit of removing the disease surgically.

Vanessa consented to the surgery. Her abdomen was opened and the surgeon removed as much tissue as he could. He took multiple samples from different areas for biopsies. Surprisingly, he could not find any visible cancer. In fact, none of the biopsies came back positive for cancer! Did that mean Vanessa didn't have cancer?

No. It showed that Vanessa had a dramatic response to chemotherapy, and any cancer that was left was visible only at a microscopic level.

Absence of evidence is not evidence of absence.

Was the surgery really necessary? In hindsight, no. But at that time, it felt like a good idea and it also was reassuring to confirm the dramatic response to chemotherapy. The surgery was tough for her. In fact she felt that with each surgery she was handling the aftereffects even worse.

"You are talking about something that has opened me up maybe 8-9 inches long. It takes 6 to 10 weeks for the healing process, for the pain to go away, the tenderness, the incision to completely close. And even months after that, it feels like a rope inside where it has been whipped, closed. Like if you were to take two pieces of material and then whip the ends and pull it tight. That's what happens to your skin. It doesn't feel flat. It feels like there is rope inside. And it stays that way for a long time," she says.

"This was the second time that I was opened up and your skin...as you get older your skin isn't as tight, so there were hernias where it didn't want to stay together. [The surgeon] wanted to put in a mesh, it is kind of like a mesh that would make it stronger so that it wouldn't herniate again. Unfortunately, when you put foreign objects in the body you are at higher risk for infection. So I ended up with this incision with hernias. You could push and it wouldn't feel solid or as thick as other areas." And this was a successful surgery, without complications! Everything takes a toll on the body, no matter how smoothly it's done.

As both scans and biopsies did not reveal any sign of cancer, further chemotherapy was discontinued. Vanessa went back to her non-medication lifestyle. The plan was to follow her by clinical exams, to monitor CEA levels, and to repeat the PET scans in a few months.

In the first week of January 2006, Vanessa got sick. She vomited a few times, but just as quickly as she had caught it, the sickness went away. A week later it happened again. Then a third time. At first, she thought it was a 24-hour flu. These sporadic illnesses were irritating, but they were nothing compared to what she had been through, so she decided not to see her doctors about them.

In April, she took a road trip with her husband to visit her daughter in Oregon. On the way back, Vanessa suddenly felt a violent burst of nausea. She opened the glove compartment and pulled out a box full of ziplock bags. She grabbed one and threw up into it. Andrew pulled over to the side of the road.

Vanessa had come down with the "flu" again, but it was more severe than before. She was rattled and couldn't stop vomiting. Andrew cleared space in the back so she could lie down for the rest of the road trip. By the time they got back home she had used up all the ziplock bags. They traced back their steps to see if there was a meal that could be causing the problem, since it seemed like she had food poisoning. However, the length of the sickness was obviously indicating something else. But by the end of the day, she no longer felt warm and nauseated. After all those hours of feeling sick in the car, she suddenly felt fine.

In the context of this story, it might seem odd that she didn't immediately run to her physician. This is a woman with an unusual, chronic colon cancer who had already demonstrated heightened (and warranted) suspicion of recurrence under more benign conditions. She had already panicked at less alarming signs. And here, she is fluctuating rapidly between highs and lows with no explanation. Why on earth didn't she contact her doctor?

"This is not that unusual. Often patients don't want to believe that their cancer is coming back—they are often afraid that if they go to their doctor, he may tell them that their cancer has come back, so they simply wait and will come in only when their symptoms become extreme," says her oncologist.

Two weeks later, as Andrew and Vanessa were exiting a Home Depot, they ran into her oncologist. He asked her how she had been doing. She sheepishly mentioned the sporadic bouts of vomiting. He told her to come by the office the next day. X-rays were taken. They didn't show anything. But her physician did suggest the possibility of a blockage in her bowels. If you think of the gastrointestinal tract as a long tube, then blocking it will cause a backup. This is what causes the vomiting. Sometimes these changes may not show up on X-rays at an early stage. At this point, you should be noticing the abundant limits in the available technologies, especially as they pertain to poor Vanessa.

The hope with a partial bowel blockage is that whatever is causing the obstruction will resolve on its own. And sometimes this would happen, as Vanessa's nausea would disappear and she would periodically feel fine. Her scans continued to look normal. But the real question was: Why was this happening? There were two likely culprits for Vanessa. Cancer, if it has regrown can obviously cause an obstruction. But the most likely factor was Vanessa's surgical history. Surgeries cause scar tissue. Her abdomen was filled with scar tissue that could block her bowels. In severe cases, ironically, surgery is performed to remove the blockage. Vanessa's situation was clinically mild. But as the year went on, her symptoms only increased.

"By the time I got into May and June I was getting sick and having stomach cramps all the time. I was having trouble eating, and I was so tired of being sick, my mind said don't eat. [That was] in June," she remembers.

This was startling to her for one reason.

"First of all, I have always had a weight problem. It is not that I like to eat a lot—it is just that I like the wrong things. I still have a weight problem," she chuckles. "I got to the point where my brain and body were so tired of vomiting that it didn't want food anymore. Literally it was like having anorexia. I mean I couldn't believe that I could ever get to the point where food sounded terrible. I tried forcing myself. I could have gone without nothing. My brain just shut off the hunger, because I was so afraid of throwing up."

And she means that. With the exception of maybe a cup of noodles, Vanessa had stopped eating. The human body can actually subsist on such a weak diet for a long time. However, it ultimately catches up with you. The real danger came in August, when she realized she could no longer drink liquids anymore. Obviously she could still physically stick water and food into her mouth. But her body rejected it. Even if she just had a small cup of water, she would vomit right after.

Having been weakened so much, Vanessa was hospitalized. A CT scan showed complete bowel blockage. She was checked in on a Saturday and needed surgery as soon as possible.

Unfortunately the local surgeons who were familiar with Vanessa were unavailable. The oncological surgeon who had performed her 2004 operation was out of town on vacation.

The other surgeon was dealing with a family issue. "His son fell off the monkey bars at a playground and he was at home taking care of him, so I had to wait till Wednesday for the surgery," she laughs, remembering the absurdity of the situation.

While she waited, she had a small tube inserted through her nose into her stomach. This is called a naso-gastric tube (naso means nose; gastric means stomach) and the purpose of this tube is to suck out air that accumulates in the stomach, to help relieve the abdominal distention and also to give rest to the intestine. Several days of this NG tube gave her minor relief. Vanessa needed that surgery. Five days after being hospitalized, she was taken into the operating room.

Forty-eight hours later, Vanessa was lying in her hospital bed, talking with her husband. She was able to eat and drink once again. The surgeon came in. "I'm afraid I have some bad news," he told her. During the operation they found cancer tissue. The surgery and the news, unfortunately, would be only the beginning of a five-month period of hell for her.

She needed to go back to chemotherapy. Remember, she had to recuperate from the surgery first. When she had rested enough,

Vanessa restarted her previous chemotherapy regimen, FOLFIRI. Soon after restarting treatment, Vanessa began to notice problems in her left leg. It felt heavy, and it took a lot of energy, or at least more than she was used to, in order to move it off the floor. On December 6th, Vanessa left the house to grocery shop. On the way to the store, she noticed that her left foot felt dense. As she walked inside the grocery store, she realized she couldn't place any weight on it. She leaned on the grocery cart, bought her food, and came back home. In agonizing pain, she laid down. She unrolled her pants and looked at her leg. It had swollen up. Not just the foot. The thigh, the calf, the ankle, the entire leg had become engorged. Vanessa had developed a blood clot in her leg.

One of the effects of cancer is that it often thickens a person's blood. Cancerous cells release chemicals that increase viscosity. With thicker blood, there is a higher chance that a person can form a blood clot. Why did it cause pain and swelling? Think of the arteries and veins as tiny streams inside your body, carrying blood to and from the various tissues. And just like when a dam obstructs the flow of water, a clot in the blood will cause overflow of fluid around the obstruction site, meaning that because the clot was in her left leg, the fluid in that left leg would leak out from the "stream" and cause a swelling.

Vanessa and her husband were advised to go to the emergency room. With a clot, the main fear is that part of the clot can shake loose, travel further along the body, and get stuck in the lungs. If multiple clots (or one big one) get stuck in the lung, people can suddenly die from lack of oxygen. So blood clots in the lung are medical emergencies.

Vanessa was admitted to the hospital and she had a filter inserted into her inferior vena cava. The inferior vena cava is one of the two major veins returning blood to the heart and blood clots will usually pass through it if they are making their way to the lungs. The filter will act as a sieve that will catch clots but allow blood to flow through. The other part of her treatment was to thin the blood itself. There are several medications that can do this but the most common long-term anti-coagulation (anti-blood clot) medication is called Coumadin, also known as Warfarin.

Unfortunately, blood thinners don't dissolve a blood clot. The medication simply reduces chances of the clot from becoming larger or breaking off. Both the filter and Coumadin are preventive measures. The clot gradually dissolved on its own, during which time Vanessa's leg remained swollen for a few months. She would constantly lie on her bed with her leg raised in the air to keep it comfortable (in this position, gravity forces extra fluids towards the rest of the body so the swelling decreases).

So Vanessa was on chemotherapy and blood thinning medications. When your body accumulates stresses, it loses the normal biomechanics that we are accustomed to. I'm talking about regular temperature, the color of the skin, breathing patterns, etc. Everything adds up. And this makes it difficult to figure out what should be happening and what is cause for concern. You look at Vanessa's hands and they are pale. Touch them and they are ice cold. "That began with the chemotherapy," she says. Her movements were static and slow—she didn't have the energy to move fast anymore.

This caused people around her to become hypersensitive to her numerous problems. "My husband was half scared to death, to the point where he drove me insane," Vanessa laughs. "If I coughed, he'd be there to ask if I'm ok. I would get up to readjust my chair and he would ask me where I'm going. I said this is a small house, Andrew—you know, where can I go, from here to the bathroom and I'm back."

One night, about a month after she was diagnosed with the blood clot, her husband noticed her eyes looked runny and her face was flushed.

"I think you have a fever," said Andrew. Vanessa disagreed. She felt different, but she didn't feel bad. And that was the barometer she used to determine how ill she was.

As Vanessa puts it, "You get to the point where you don't know what's causing you to feel bad...you can blame it on the cancer, the chemo, the back pain, you don't know what is causing what. It might have been how I normally felt. When he told me I was running a temperature, I didn't feel like I was sick, because the effects of the chemotherapy make you normally feel like you're bottoming out of energy." The thermometer didn't lie though. Vanessa had a temperature of 102 degrees Fahrenheit.

She was started on once a day IV antibiotics. Vanessa's fever didn't go away. It was back to the hospital for her. Chemotherapy had to be stopped at this point. You don't want to put a person through the side effects of chemotherapy while they are infected. In any case, chemo suppresses the immune system that one needs to fight off any infection. Vanessa was given intensive IV antibiotics in the hospital. Tests were run to find a source for her fever, but they were inconclusive.

Assuming there was an infection, the antibiotics did their job and her fever went away. Several days later, her temperature flared again. Her doctors told her that with the antibiotics, the infection was being suppressed but not being eradicated. They had to find the source. Eventually, they looked into her portacath, a device implanted underneath the skin that acts as an easy tunnel into the venous system. This is useful for chemotherapy patients because it grants instant access to the venous system for administration of chemotherapy drugs. Unfortunately, it is a device and can get infected (remember, anything that is not natural within the body can be easily contaminated by bacteria or fungus). The treatment is to remove the device. It's a simple procedure, but it was riskier for Vanessa because of the Coumadin that made it easier for her to bleed.

I've mentioned multiple times now the cumulative effect of medical treatments on the body and it was starting to show on Vanessa. She was hospitalized because of an infection. That infection was caused by the corruption of a simple medical device. That medical device was inserted to help deliver chemotherapy drugs to her. These chemo drugs in turn weakened her immune system, so when the portacath became infected she had difficulty in fighting off the infection. Meanwhile, her blood had been thickened by the cancer that caused dangerous blood clots, but the drugs used to keep it thin had to be stopped so she could safely take out the device causing a life-threatening infection. Do you see how complicated the process of treatment can become?

Vanessa had a protracted stay in the hospital. It took three weeks in the hospital before she was declared infection-free. A new portacath was inserted so that she could renew her chemotherapy treatment. This was late February 2007, just two and a half months after her blood clot incident. Her leg was still swollen and at night she was forced to rest it on a tower of pillows.

Within a month though, Vanessa was back in the hospital. Her fever had returned along with severe chills, vomiting, and diarrhea. The doctors checked the new portacath but there was no problem with it. In fact, the infection was a completely new bug.

Her stool showed evidence of a toxin-producing bacteria called Clostridium Difficile, also known as C. Diff.

Before I explain this infection, you should understand that not all bacteria are bad for humans. In fact there are plenty of good bacteria that keep people healthy. C. Diff is a bacteria that exists inside every person's intestines. The reason it does not normally cause an infection is that it is kept in check by good bacteria that also reside in every person's bowels.

Now, consider what happens when a person takes an antibiotic. Antibiotics are not specific for just one type of bacteria. They travel throughout the body and can destroy multiple types of bacteria, including the ones causing an infection but also helpful bacteria . This is similar to what happens in chemotherapy, where the drug that is used to kill rapidly dividing cancer cells also destroys any other cell that rapidly divides. If a person has been on lengthy doses of antibiotics, there is a strong possibility the good bacteria can be wiped out. Once this happens, the checkpoint that keeps C. Diff from proliferating disappears, and you can develop a C. Difficile infection.

The danger with this bacteria is that it releases a toxin and when its numbers increase so does the amount of toxin. Ironically, the solution to this problem is more antibiotics. Vanessa was started on one called vancomycin. One of vancomycin's unique properties is that if taken orally it's not absorbed well by the body. This means if it is given by mouth it goes into your digestive tract and basically stays there instead of going into the blood stream. This concentrates its effect in the gastrointestinal tract and allows it to target the C. Diff..

And while there was a solution to each immediate issue, the real problem was that these hospitalizations were interfering with her chemo treatments (as in she couldn't receive them until she was stable). The cancer wasn't waiting around for Vanessa to recover from her fevers.

As she fought off the infection, she noticed a strange tightness in her left abdomen. Day by day it became bulkier. She pointed it out to her physician while she was in the hospital. He pressed a finger to it. It was hard as a rock. A CT scan showed a new 19 cm area "collection" around her left kidney. The physicians immediately knew it wasn't a tumor. Her history had shown her colon cancer to be slow-growing and this had developed in days. It was either fluid secreted by the cancer, a collection of blood (hematoma), or a collection of pus (an abscess). A needle was inserted into her abdomen and pus came out. I'll cover how this even started in just a bit.

There were several different options. Doctors could have gone in and surgically removed the whole mass at that point. But again, these invasive procedures have a cumulative effect on the body and it's preferable to avoid them when possible. Her physicians opted for using a small drainage catheter (tube) that was inserted into the wound. This catheter was attached to a small bag so the liquid inside the abscess would continuously empty into it. Vanessa was asked to take a bottle of saline solution and squirt it into the catheter. By flooding the abscess cavity with the saline solution, the infected liquid inside would be pushed out into the bag.

Vanessa was sent back home with this makeshift apparatus attached. It had to stay in the same place at all times and at night her husband would have to empty the bag of its disgusting thick, yellow contents.

Unfortunately, a week and a half after she had been discharged home, her abdomen again increased in size. "It didn't make any sense," said Vanessa. "Every night the bag kept filling up with fluid. My gut kept expanding."

She was readmitted back into the hospital on April 30th 2007. She was also suffering from constant diarrhea at that point.

Amazingly enough, she tested positive for C. Difficile again. Vancomycin was restarted. She also had a larger drain inserted into the abscess. And even then her abdomen continued to expand. That's an amazing feat, if you think about it. The infection created fluid at a fast enough rate so that it not only maintained balance with the amount being forced out, but also created an excess supply.

The physicians had tried to avoid a major surgical procedure, however there was no other choice but to go in.

As Vanessa later put it, "That was the worst surgery I've gone through."

When the surgeons opened her up, they found a wall of infection enclosing her left kidney. So let's explore the confluence of factors that created this disaster.

In 2000, Vanessa had found out that her left kidney was no longer functioning. Since everyone is blessed with two kidneys this was not an issue, and a decision was made to just leave it in her. Since the "dead" kidney was not doing her any harm, it did not make any sense to do a major surgical procedure to remove it. But when an organ stops working, the blood supply to that tissue can diminish over time. If that happens, then the tissue actually starts to die (just because it was not functioning doesn't mean the kidney's cells died). If a tissue dies it's more likely to become infected.

So that was the first problem; the kidney had become infected.

The next problem stemmed from Vanessa's hospital visits over the past few months. They had interfered with her chemotherapy treatments. During this time, the cancer continued to grow. In fact, it had collected around the kidney. Because dead tissue doesn't absorb medicine well (chemotherapy travels through the bloodstream, and if there is no blood supply to a tissue then it doesn't get affected by the medicine), the area around the kidney had begun to collect cancer cells. As a result, Vanessa had an infected dead kidney with a large amount of cancer cells around it.

The third issue came from all her surgeries. Wounds create scars. The bigger the wound, the more scar tissue you have. Vanessa had gone through several major procedures at this point, and each created a large amount of scar tissue. In addition, opening up the abdomen exposes it to the outside environment; that is a risk factor for infection in itself. All these factors contributed to the giant bulk inside her abdomen that the doctors had to remove.

Do you see how ailments and treatments can compound other issues?

To sum up, within the last five months Vanessa had suffered a debilitating blood clot in her left leg, five major fevers including two bouts of C. Difficile infection, and an abscess that required major surgery. To say the least, that's a taxing medical history. And yet, the cancer continued to grow because Vanessa was obliged to stay off the chemotherapy to treat other problems. Vanessa wouldn't restart the chemo until September 9th, 2007, nearly nine months after she had discontinued it.

First, she had to recover from the surgery. With the type of incision her surgeons had made, they could not close her up. It needed to heal up from the inside. She had the surgery in May and her wound didn't close until August. That meant she had an opening in her left torso for over three months!

"What they do, it's almost a Clorox type of solution … actually you can do it with Clorox and water. They had my husband insert gauze (covered in solution) into the incision and what it does is draw out any infection and gunk out of it. It very slowly, from the inside out, closes. Very slowly, over two or three weeks, you notice you have to use less of the gauze. It is all sterile. You have to wear gloves and you have to use these sterile solutions to make it and it hurts putting it in. It kind of stings. It's like alcohol. You put alcohol in a wound and it burns. I had an abdominal pad, thick and square, after he shoved the gauze in there he would tape the abdominal pad. He'd have to rip the tape off at some point to redo it. We're not talking about a couple of days. We are talking about day after day."

To add insult to injury, Vanessa became allergic to the adhesive on the tape and the skin around the wound puffed up and began to tear from the constant application and removal of it.

Her CEA was 209. Back in January it was 35. You don't get rest from these battles. The problems don't wait to be resolved one by one. Physically she was slow to recuperate, but mentally she was struggling as well. During those periods when Vanessa wasn't shackled to a hospital bed, she lay at home knowing her cancer was spreading and hoping she could recover fast enough to go to war with it again.

By the time she resumed her chemotherapy at the end of 2007, there was evidence of cancer in her lungs, liver, and even the bones. But as before, her chemotherapy regimen reduced the cancer load. She was started on a relatively new drug, Avastin, which works by cutting off the blood supply to cancer and therefore starves the growing cancer cells. On its own it is relatively ineffective, but in combination with chemotherapy it can help significantly in killing cancer cells. However, it does not eradicate the cancer. It just buys more time with minimal side effects.-

Fast-forward to 2010. Almost fifteen years after being declared cancer-free, Vanessa was still on her chemotherapy treatments. Because her cancer continued to progress, she started on a new drug called Erbitux, part of a new class of drugs called Targeted Therapy. These drugs specifically target proteins in cancer cells and kill them with many fewer side effects than chemotherapy. Targeted therapy works best when given in combination with chemotherapy. Vanessa had a very good response, as suggested by a dramatic improvement in her quality of life and a decreased CEA. The initial response was short-lived, as a scan showed cancer resurgence after several months. It would be the pattern of her health and treatment from there on out. It's endless.

Such a long journey – was it worth it?

"I think you have to try and remain positive. You don't all the time. I don't all the time. There are some times I think it would be a whole lot easier if there was no one depending on me to survive, because it'd be a lot easier to give up. But then I think back and I think that I'm not ready to die. I have lived long enough to see my daughter graduate from high school- which I didn't think initially I'd see- from college, get married, and have my grandson. I never dreamt I would live long enough to see this. You ask whether or not this is worth it, and it is. I still get sick after chemotherapy, but not all the time. I still go through periods of time where I say can I keep doing this and other periods where I say I hope I can do this so long as I can survive. You need to strive to retain as much of what is normal to you as you can. It takes a lot of support from family," Vanessa explains.

"If it was only me, I don't think I would have pushed as long as I have. I still feel like I have a long time yet to go. There are peaks and valleys. Sometimes things look good like right now, and I may have to go off chemo for a while, and you never know where you will reach that point where there is nothing left for them to do. But there is always hope with these new drugs."

Vanessa's case was highly unusual. Her cancer was more stubborn than originally predicted. To think that in 1993 she was told that as long as she survived five years without cancer recurrence she could rest easy! Her cancer was growing slowly enough so new medications kept popping up which offered mild salvation. None could completely cure her. Her life span was unpredictable, but it was limited. Eventually the cancer would win. As late as August 2011 Vanessa was still receiving intermittent chemotherapy. She had cancer at multiple sites in the bones. She needed radiation therapy to the spine to control pain. Her chemotherapy options were limited, as she had progressed through all available medications and other options for colon cancer. Because of her poor health, she was not considered a candidate for clinical trials.

Post Script: She died later that year, seventeen years after the initial diagnosis and ten years after the first signs of relapse.

Her oncologist remarks, "Vanessa was a remarkable woman. Tough, salt of the earth type. She had one complication after another and was often quite miserable, but she rarely complained. When she complained I knew there was some significant issue and always listened to her. She got fired from her job for the 'crime' of getting a complicated cancer, her HMO gave her a tough time as if it was her fault for getting a cancer; throughout all this she remained stoic and never seemed bitter. Despite all her travails she remained grateful that her life could be prolonged so many years and she could see her family grow and a grandchild be born. She always verbally thanked me and my staff despite being in pain and discomfort. I don't think I will ever forget her and what she went through."

It's (Not) Textbook

"I'M VERY ANGRY at what happened," Karen says. She pauses as she tries to calm down. She wants to express her thoughts more delicately. "I'm angry because the doctor missed the diagnosis. The skin doctor missed it....[We asked him] what is going on here. And he said 'It's fine.' It's fine?! He should have rechecked the margins, something else should have been done."

She stops again. She looks like she wants to say more, but she restrains herself. I ask her if she was upset because the doctor made a mistake, or because she thinks he didn't put enough effort into helping her husband, Peter.

Another pause. She shakes her head slightly. Karen has a good reason to cut off her answer. "It was missed. He missed it. He obviously did not get all the tumor out...it was obviously deeper than he thought. Whether I'm wrong or not...whether I'm right or not....I've put it out of my mind."

She has not. "I just let it go now. Peter is alive and well, so that's all—*but it was missed by him*," she finishes emphatically.

Her reaction is normal. Despite her best efforts to hide it, her thoughts may as well be stamped onto her forehead. Peter also believes his wife is still angry at their dermatologist. What is more interesting, though, is why she is so hesitant to criticize the dermatologist in public: he and her husband are colleagues. Peter is a practicing cardiologist.

We're going to take a look at Peter's battle with cancer because it intertwines with a sensitive issue for many patients: knowledge. We have always had an innate desire to understand the conditions that affect our health. That desire is only magnified by the severity of the ailment. Through the internet and resources such as WebMD, patients have more access than ever before to a variety of sources outlining medical conditions and treatment options.

Does it help, though? Forget for a moment the trouble of actually obtaining accurate information, which can be quite difficult. What happens if you do obtain the proper facts? I can read all I want about how to construct a car or sculpt a statue, but putting it into practice is an entirely different matter. When the layperson reads information about a disease, how practical is it? Can you catch things your doctors miss? Can you alert them to new breakthroughs they aren't aware of?

Perhaps it resolves the dilemma of choice. Patients are constantly given multiple options on how to deal with their disease. Each choice comes with pros and cons. In the medical world, it is seen as a benefit derived from medicine's advancement. We pat ourselves on the back for allowing patients to be independent. They get to participate in their healthcare. But it can be agonizing to make these decisions! Patients constantly ask their doctor, "What would you do in my shoes?" It stands to reason that if patients were knowledgeable enough, they wouldn't need to ask their physicians to help them choose.

Peter, a physician, and Karen, an ICU nurse, collectively have more knowledge of cancer and the operations and treatments involved in the battle with disease than most patients ever will. We're going to see how a physician deals with cancer when they are in the patient's chair. We're going to examine whether that knowledge is beneficial. We might even see times when it could be harmful.

Peter has been practicing medicine in northern California for over twenty-five years. In 2007, he was diagnosed with a squamous cell cancer. What followed was an utter disaster.

Karen shows me photos of her husband, taken years before, on her locker. I met Peter recently and he didn't look the same as he does in the color prints.

It might have been the weight. "He used to be 240 pounds, but now he's at about 190," Karen says. That's a muscular 240, not an obese 240. Peter used to be a weightlifter, but he was forced to take a break from that hobby for several-years.

It might be the hair. He has a full head in the photo, but now he is thinning to bald.

It could be the droop I saw in the left side of Peter's face. It is a condition that will never completely resolve. I was told that it's not as striking as it used to be. Still, the portrait of him that you see in the waiting room of his office is decidedly different from the image you see when you greet him at the front door. His left lips are stiff, his cheek taut, and his eye looks as if it is always on the cusp of sliding down.

I think it's something else though. I think it's a matter of presence.

Before I explain, there are a few things that you need to know about Peter. The first factor to consider is that he is a doctor. Yes, I've already mentioned what he does for a living. But more than just being his occupation, he has the old-school stereotypical doctor's personality. Stoic, doesn't like to complain, works long hours, used to making decisions, and is a man of few words (and yes, this is why Karen is quoted so much in the story). He's tall, and having lifted weights for so long he is physically dominating. In short, this is a man who creates initial impressions of strength. But it's been diminished. I don't think he's as imposing as he used to be.

Peter was born in Modesto, California and moved to Phoenix and later Mississippi, where he spent much of his childhood. Most of the time he worked on the family farm. For college, he returned to Arizona (Arizona State University) and then went to medical school at the University of Arizona. Finally, he moved back to Modesto to set up his clinical practice. That's a pretty quick sketch of his early years, but it already gives us some good information when it comes to skin cancer.

First, we see that Peter grew up in areas with sunny climates. His farm work also meant that he would be outside for long periods of time. So he's had lots of sun exposure. Being Caucasian, he has pale skin and thus is at increased risk for skin changes due to the sun's rays. There are three major types of skin cancer: squamous cell, basal cell, and melanomas.

How do they occur? How is it that the sun, a natural source of life and energy, could be implicated in cancer? Unfortunately, while the sun is necessary for life on earth, overexposure to it causes problems. Specifically, there is something called UV radiation in sunlight. The energy in that UV radiation is a type that can directly alter or mutate DNA. As we explained in Mike's story, these mutations affect cells, causing them to keep replicating or eliminate their innate abilities to terminate replication. As the human race is exposed to the sun all the time, it understandably takes an enormous amount of radiation to cause enough mutations for cancer growth. Often you will see precursors to an actual cancer. Peter, for example was used to seeing skin changes called "actinic keratosis" on his body.

Actinic keratosis are small, darkened scaly patches of skin. Although they are not harmful on their own, they have the ability to convert into a skin cancer. The best way to treat them is by removing these patches. They can also be cauterized (burned), or frozen. As they can mimic or convert into a skin cancer, check-ups are extremely important. Almost every six months, some new skin mark would appear and Peter would have it checked by his dermatologist. This cycle continued until 2007 when a biopsy of one of Peter's numerous skin lesions came up positive for squamous cell cancer. This actually wasn't a source of concern.

Let's pause right there and examine that statement. Pretend you have little to zero knowledge of cancers. Anything you do know has been acquired through anecdotes or the occasional mention of it on the news or from friends who know everything about anything. Your conception of malignancy is similar to the average person: it is a devastating disease that kills many people. Your life is quite stress-free until one day you notice a small lesion on your chin. Who knows how long it's been there; perhaps it is has been a very recent development. You book an appointment with a physician. You're a bit nervous as they examine and biopsy it. A week later you return to the office. You're told that you have a squamous cell carcinoma. You have cancer. You panic and immediately start to wonder how long you have to live. The physician stops you mid-panic to tell you that it is actually a very harmless cancer. You have nothing to be worried about. You brush off the reassurance, but it is actually true. Squamous cell skin cancer is very common and easy to treat. It has a mortality rate of less than 0.3%.

However, the real question is: Do the statistics alleviate your fear? Do the facts neutralize the perception of the word cancer? It's an important question, because Peter's reaction to his diagnosis played a great role in his future. As a medical professional, he was so thoroughly accustomed to medical statistics and the absolute truth they provide in most diseases that he reacted to the squamous cell cancer with nonchalance. It was not a big deal to him.

He had probably seen multitudes of people diagnosed with it who had uneventful treatments. Even in medical school it is hammered into the aspiring physician's brain that squamous cell carcinoma of the skin is not something to worry about. And for the most part, it never is. But the layperson doesn't know that. And even if they knew the statistic it probably wouldn't matter. They're fighting a battle against their own perception. Truth has little potency in this matter.

Squamous cell skin cancer is usually easy to treat. The skin lesion just needs to be removed. The key is to make sure the margins are clear. The term clear margins means the edges of the specimen excised do not have any cancer cells, thereby indicating that no cancer cells are left behind and the cancer has been removed completely. Think about it. Cancer, until it spreads, is contained in one big group. You don't want to leave a single cancer cell in the skin, because it has the ability to replicate indefinitely and will cause problems down the line. So once you note that you have reached normal skin cell lining in every direction from the cancerous lesion that's removed, you've theoretically neutered the malignancy for good.

The procedure is minor surgery. A small incision is made, and based on the estimates for margins, an area is removed from the skin. Peter's cancer happened to be on the left side of his face, near the edge of his jawline.

That should have been the end of the story. As Karen puts it, "So he had a spot removed, no big deal. It was a squamous cell cancer, no big deal. They took it out, cleared the margin. Didn't think much of it."

Several months later, Peter woke up one morning with what felt like a toothache. He shrugged it off, but the next day it was still there. Strangely, he couldn't tell if it was actually coming from the teeth.

Karen remembers it vividly only because Peter's reaction was so unusual. "I saw him, after I came back home from working, taking Tylenol. I thought that was strange. All he ever took was a blood pressure medication in the morning," she remembers.

She approached him to see if everything was alright.

"My face is hurting," Peter said as he pre-empted her question. It was happening right at the spot where he had the squamous cell cancer removed. On Karen's suggestion, he decided to go back to the dermatologist to get it checked out. The dermatologist examined him, but could not find anything of concern. "Not related to the cancer; the margins were clear," he reassured Peter.

So Peter didn't think it was the cancer. Fair enough, since he had just gotten a clean bill of health from the dermatologist. Faith in the system, in statistics, was reigning paramount here. But again, imagine if it's you in his position. You had a cancer removed on the left side of your face and then a couple of months later you start to get pain...in the left side of the face. How would you react?

Peter was confident the pain would resolve. It did not go away, though. Several weeks later, Peter woke up feeling a strange sensation in his face. He ignored it and began his normal morning routine. While he was toweling himself off after the shower, he looked in the mirror for the first time that morning and noticed his left eye looked different. It had a slight droop, as if the eye had begun to slide down. Initially, this didn't alarm either him or Karen too much.

"I figured you know, he has stress in his job, and whenever he gets really stressed he gets a numb lip, and this would happen once or twice a year. It would last for a few days and then it would go away, and now you start looking at the possible reasons for a face droop. It is either a tumor, or something is there, or it is stress. So I figured it was stress," Karen recalls.

"I'm not stressed," Peter told her as he rejected her theory. He repeated the words several more times so she got the message. He took Advil and Prednisone, drugs that reduce inflammation in the body. If it were a stress reaction, the drugs would alleviate the symptom. Days went by, and the droop didn't go away. It became more pronounced. Peter booked an appointment with a neurologist, who gave him a diagnosis of Bell's palsy.

Bell's palsy is the most common cause of a facial droop. It is caused by a viral infection that inflames the facial nerve. Nerves can act like power cords to the muscles of the body. Though we don't think about the face having muscles, it does. Whenever you raise your eyebrows or smile or bite down, the muscles of the face control these actions. The facial nerve is an important nerve responsible for activating many of the muscles in the face. When it is damaged, it can no longer activate those muscles. Thus, instead of the face staying taut as it does normally, it starts to droop.

Treatment with steroids and anti-viral drugs often leads to rapid improvement in the vast majority of cases (90%) and the condition usually vanishes without a trace.

But there was something else to consider. Nerves control more than muscles; they also relay sensations (including pain). From a biological point of view, it wouldn't make sense for one nerve to control action and also act as a sensory monitor. Thus, there are nerves for the roles of sensation and others for movement. The facial nerve controls the muscle of the face, but doesn't relay sensation from the face. Another nerve, called the trigeminal nerve, takes care of that function. Bell's palsy usually spares the trigeminal nerve. Because of that, a person shouldn't have pain in Bell's palsy. And in fact, pain is rarely reported with the diagnosis.

So why was Peter having pain?

It's an important nuance that could easily be missed if you haven't seen the disease. If you read about it in a textbook what you would most likely pick up are major facets such as the facial droop, how long it lasts, etiology, and treatment—not "trivial" details like pain.

Just like any other patient (or family member of a patient) in this situation, Karen set about researching the disease. Although Peter and she knew of Bell's palsy and understood it, they weren't experts on the ailment. They didn't know all the nuances. Despite their medical knowledge, and the easy access they had to other physicians, Peter and Karen found themselves in the same situation any other patient would be in these circumstances. So they wanted to research the important difference between classic Bell's palsy and what Peter was going through: the disease usually doesn't cause pain. The key word there is usually. Karen found cases where pain had been described with Bell's palsy.

A second opinion from another neurologist did not reveal anything new. He also confirmed the diagnosis of Bell's palsy, and told them it would go away on its own. A CT scan of Peter's head was normal and reassured everyone involved in the diagnosis. But how long would Peter need to wait for it to go away? The more time that passed, the more pain he had. Likewise, the facial droop had not improved.

Still worried they were missing something, they made more appointments with the dermatologist, and each time were told there was nothing to worry about from a cancer viewpoint. Peter's pain was increasing. Even more worrisome was his resistance to pain medication. No matter how many pills he popped, the pain wouldn't go away.

"To the dermatologist, I asked if there could be a relation to the cancer. I didn't ask the neurologist that. All I knew was that I had pain and the droop. He didn't know the reason, but he knew that pain and Bell's palsy don't go together," Peter says.

He and Karen had found rare cases in neurology literature about Bell's palsy associated with pain. They used these examples to reassure themselves, but they knew something was off.

Weeks went by and the pain only increased. The droop became more exaggerated. If you've never seen Bell's palsy, you should take a moment to go look it up. It's a disturbing disease as the visual distortion is happening directly on the face.

Peter continued to work through this period. Eventually his patients began to question him about his condition. It was all in good concern, of course, but part of the physician's power is the aura of control. The doctor is supposed to know exactly what is going on, and it's unsettling when they don't. If a doctor is in bad shape himself, some of that omnipotent luster fades. When the deterioration happens to a man as alpha as Peter, it's magnified even more.

For Karen, the more worrisome problem was the change to Peter's personality. "When you are in pain, everything else in your life stops because you don't feel good. Because you don't feel good, you don't feel like doing anything," Peter explains. Peter had moved on to more potent pain medications, such as Vicodin. The pain wasn't excruciating, but it wouldn't let up, and its constant throbbing was a weight on his mind and a leech on his energy. He was becoming sedentary, a descriptor he had never been associated with.

Karen had continued to research Bell's palsy throughout this period. She found out about a medical practice, near Los Angeles, that was supposed to cure the pain of Bell's palsy. An associate professor from UCLA used acupuncture to treat the patients. "She had a radio talk show. It was like 5 star," says Karen.

It's not an insane idea. Some studies have suggested that intense acupuncture can improve Bell's palsy conditions. Peter, as stringent a devotee to Western medicine as there is, wasn't interested.

His assessment of acupuncture? "Doesn't work. It is a waste of time."

However, several months of constant pain had pushed him to the point of desperation. None of the doctors he had spoken to had any solutions for him. Why wouldn't he look for answers beyond the conventional marketplace? If Western medicine had all the answers, there wouldn't be a market for alternatives.

Peter agreed to give the clinic a shot. He and Karen traveled down to Southern California. Naturally, Peter has a pilot's license, so he flew the two of them down there (no word on rumors that he parachuted into the clinic directly).

The basis for the visit was to treat the pain through acupuncture (I was going to add an explanation of how this works, but honestly, after reading about it I still don't understand. So there.). The physician instructed Peter to lie on his back and began inserting needles into his face, and then his hands, and finally his feet. Karen watched as Peter was turned into a pincushion. With every needle, Peter felt more uncomfortable. After all the needles were in, Peter was told to stay still and let the acupuncture do its work. Finally, enough time had passed. The needles were taken out. When the last one was removed, Peter groaned and jumped out of his chair. The acupuncturist took a look at his face.

"Oh, wow, it is still crooked. You're not any better yet," she exclaimed as she looked at his eye. "Well, it will get better by tomorrow. If not, come back and we'll do it again." She advised Peter and Karen to fly down the next weekend and repeat the process.

Peter replied bluntly, "Nope."

On the flight home, the two of them laid out what they knew. "By this time we already had CT's and knew there were no tumors anywhere, so we already had that stuff done. We knew we weren't dealing with a mass at that point. I remember being so optimistic," Karen remembers.

"I don't remember anything except the flight," Peter adds.

Peter wanted no more treatments. Karen pushed him to try out the acupuncture again, this time under the hands of a local physician. "Just give it a shot," she urged him. Against his better judgment, he agreed. "Yeah, he was a lot rougher than [the UCLA physician]. All it did was make the pain worse. He wanted me to come back again as well," Peter remembers as he shook his head.

What changed his mind about doing the acupuncture?

After all, he didn't believe in it before he tried it. "Well, I still didn't understand it. I thought it might help without my understanding what it was," he explains.

Peter resigned himself to the idea that there was no cure for his disease. Five months after he first felt the pain in his cheek, the throb had pushed him to stronger narcotics and dramatically changed his facial features. What happened next was an instance where Peter's occupation helped him. One morning, as he passed through the 4th floor of his hospital, Peter ran into an ENT (ear, nose, and throat) doctor he was only slightly acquainted with.

"Peter! What happened to you?" she exclaimed as she looked at his face.

He explained the Bell's palsy he had been afflicted with. She then asked about the scar on his cheek. It was the remnant from his skin cancer removal. This was fortuitous. She had moved to town after working at the M.D. Anderson cancer center in Houston, Texas. This famous clinic is sent many of the rarest cancer cases.

"Oh, that was the squamous cell carcinoma that was taken out," he said nonchalantly. Her eyes widened.

"That's peri-neural invasion of the facial nerve!" she told him (I'll explain the diagnosis later). Every other physician in the hospital had seen Peter in passing through the past five months, and all of them had tried to figure out what was wrong. Peter had even asked the dermatologist point blank about the possibility of the cancer being responsible for the droop and the pain and he had flatly denied it. And only this chance encounter, with a colleague whom he rarely spoke to, provided the solution to Peter's problem. She asked him to bring his scans to her office, so that a colleague of theirs who was more familiar with the disease would be able to confirm it.

As I've written so far, this diagnosis was possible only through the circumstances of Peter's profession. People aren't running into doctors at the grocery store and getting diagnosed with rare ailments. In that sense, it's a blessing that Peter is a physician. But there is another side to this story. Is it possible it had taken so long to be diagnosed only because of Peter's medical knowledge?

"It's pretty reasonable that my advanced knowledge of medicine [hurt]…I don't have to go through routine care or routine evaluations…and this knowledge may have impeded me from seeking specialist help," Peter admits.

Yes, he had sought the help of his peers, but given the severity of symptoms, this seems like rather a meek effort. Understanding the normal etiology of his symptoms seemed to relieve Peter, perhaps a bit too much. It's difficult to Monday morning quarterback the situation, given how many physicians had missed the diagnosis. Then again, perhaps the layperson heads directly to a university center more familiar with these rare cases. A component of fear is mystery. Peter didn't have this fear of his squamous cell carcinoma because he understood it so well. Shrugging it off was a natural, although possibly harmful reaction.

But why do situations like this occur? Why don't patients always get answers when they exist? There are always two possibilities as to why a patient has not received good counsel. The first—the more depressing and yet absolutely acceptable explanation—is that science has not evolved to the point where an answer can be provided. The second reason, infuriating and frustrating, is the physician missed the diagnosis because of ignorance or simply not bothering to research it further.

Would patient knowledge help with the second? It's possible, albeit highly unlikely.

If Peter is upset about how it played out, he doesn't show it. "My attitude toward them missing it....My wife was really pissed. I wasn't. I was disappointed. But I also understood it was very rare and could be missed easily. My thinking was that was just the way things work. If I weren't a physician, it wouldn't have gotten picked up at all; it would have been missed totally. Both the dermatologist and neurologist I went to are respected in their fields and both missed it. Unless someone was lucky enough to go to the right person at the right time, I would have died from it," he says.

Peter was quite fortunate that it was diagnosed relatively early. The peri-neural invasion would have been caught eventually but for the wrong reasons. "More neurological symptoms would have popped up and eventually a diagnosis would have been made. But see the problem with a peri-neural invasion is that it travels along the nerve sheath and travels peripherally to the brain stem. And once it gets to the brain stem, it is all over. But until it gets to the brain stem you don't get any new neurological symptoms. So you know you're toast at that point," Peter explains. The brain stem is a vital part of the central nervous system and controls necessary actions like breathing. Like the brain, it is a delicate structure and easy to injure. And if the cancer reaches that area, there is nothing in the medical field that can treat it. Surgery won't be able to remove it; chemo and radiation will be far too damaging to the area.

Peter went to see the other ENT doctor. His history was highly suggestive of peri-neural invasion of the facial nerve. This is a rare occurrence, an exacerbation of uncontained squamous cell carcinoma. Let's assume the resection of the cancer had not been complete. Malignant cells were still deep in the skin tissue after the surgery. Being cancer cells, they replicated over and over, and at some point they were able to break through the superficial part of the face and go even deeper. In fact, they began to spread into the area surrounding the facial nerve. Either through their own bulk or the inflammation they cause, these malignant cells would interfere with the facial nerve. This caused Peter's facial droop. They could also affect other nerves in the area. The head, because it has such tiny volume with strict constraints to space, is very sensitive to volume change. Thus any growth deep to the layers of the skin is going to cause pain.

Although Peter's history pointed to this diagnosis, the only way for his physicians to know for sure would be to biopsy the facial nerve itself. Unfortunately, given the anatomy of the face, the only way to biopsy the facial nerve would be to open up the face.

It's a bit difficult to understand the minutiae of this surgery without seeing a picture of all the structures of the face, but if you did look at one you would immediately notice how complicated and intricate it is. And what should be obvious is how easy it would be to disrupt vital nerves, blood vessels, muscles, etc. of the face during surgery. Although this is always a possibility during any surgery, there is certainly more leeway when dealing with a larger space such as the abdomen.

This all might seem obvious, but it is vital to consider and we'll see its importance when we consider the options offered to Peter by his physicians. He agreed to the biopsy. It was positive for the squamous cell cancer. It required more major surgeries. By 2008, Peter had undergone a left total parotidectomy (removal of the parotid gland). The parotid gland is one of three salivary glands that, as their name suggests, provide saliva. As far as anatomy goes, the facial nerve travels through the parotid gland, almost bisecting it. In each and every one of these surgeries, the tissue that must be removed is also delicately intertwined with vital nerves and vasculature. There is a balance between the amount of malignant tissue that can be removed and the amount of damage the surgeons are willing to cause to surrounding structures.

The numerous surgeries had altered Peter's look far beyond the distortion of the facial palsy. "It was ugly," says Karen. Peter did not want to walk around with a giant gash on his face, and so the surgeons sutured dressings to the skin. Soon after, in the month of October, Peter returned to work. In celebration of Halloween, Karen taped a plastic spider onto his dressing that Peter gleefully paraded throughout the hospital.

Shortly after his third surgery, while he was still confined to his bed, the surgeons visited Peter. They wanted to see if any neurological damage had been caused by the operation itself. It's easy during such surgeries to injure one of the numerous nerves coursing through the face. Peter was asked to raise his eyebrows, puff out his cheeks, and wiggle his nose – anything that could demonstrate he had full control and power over all the muscles of the face. He was unable to wrinkle his forehead, close his eyes, wiggle his nose, and even unable to move his lower left lip. The facial nerve wasn't working at full capacity. Whether that was due to direct injury or indirect injury through processes like inflammation could never be determined. There was an immense pain in the left side of his face, at the temporal-mandibular joint (think of that as the corner of the jawline, below the ears).

To make matters worse, there were still cancer cells left inside his face. The surgeons had taken out as much tissue as they dared, but they had run into a situation they were not comfortable with.

This has nothing to do with the skill of the surgeon, and more about their experience with the type of surgery. While his doctors were comfortable with the initial operations, they soon realized the disease was advanced and would require an expertise they did not have.

Peter, on the advice of the ENT physician and several of his colleagues, booked an appointment with a surgeon at Stanford who was well acquainted with metastasized facial cancers. After reviewing Peter's file, he came up with a plan: he and his team would open up Peter's face once again and operate down the path of the facial nerve. This meant that a pathologist would be present during the operation and would examine every removed section of tissue under microscope as the surgery was ongoing. They would start near the beginning of the facial nerve and work their way to where it finished in the brain stem. Afterwards they would begin Peter on chemotherapy and radiation.

It should be apparent, especially when compared to the details of Peter's previous surgery, that this would be a massive undertaking. Once again, pretend you're in his shoes. You're being told by an expert at Stanford Medical Center, one of the most prestigious hospitals in the country, that you need this surgery in order to maximize your chance to live. You've already been exhausted by previous surgeries that have left you unable to feel the top of your lip, express certain emotions on your face, and certainly affected its aesthetic quality. This new surgery will worsen all of that. You can read whatever information is out there, but at this point there will be few, if any, resources to detail the chances of success, and no standardized recommendations. In other words, you are in a gray zone of medicine. You can, of course, refuse. But would you want to? Especially after going through everything else? Doesn't that seem like a waste?

Peter and Karen spent the days after the Stanford meeting debating their next course of action. Peter had initially agreed with the doctor's approach. The more he thought about it, though, the less he wanted to go through with it. He was worn out. He couldn't fathom how he was going to recover from a surgery of that magnitude.

He called the Stanford physician and told him about his concerns. He was told to get a third opinion. So Peter went across the bay, to the University of California, San Francisco medical center. A surgical oncologist reviewed his file.

"No more surgery," he told Peter. "You can't keep cutting away at something you can't even see. You need radiation and chemotherapy and all you're doing is wasting time."

So, a *slightly* different approach than what Stanford's specialist had recommended. Multiple things to consider here, but the two most important are:

1) How is it possible for two specialists to look at the same exact data and offer completely opposite viewpoints?

2) When two specialists are offering opposite viewpoints, how do you make the right choice?

To answer the first question, I spoke to his oncologist, who said, "This does not happen very often, but can happen if the problem and situation is uncommon. Most decisions are made based on doing the same thing again and again; data is collected and based on the data, recommendations are made, so they generally tend to be quite uniform. Unfortunately, some problems are rare and unusual, so opinions can be quite different. As Peter's case was unusual, data based on repeated treatment of his condition are not available. We do know that in this case cancer cells were left behind, as suggested by the positive margins. So the question was: for the microscopic disease left behind, is surgery plus chemotherapy plus radiation therapy necessary, or is chemotherapy and radiation therapy alone, without surgery, sufficient? This was the dilemma, so now decisions need to be based on personal experience, physician biases, and patient preference. In these situations there is no right or wrong answer, but it's just a matter of making a decision."

The second question unfortunately is impossible to answer. Consider the difficulty of Peter's decision here. Stanford and UCSF are two of the most renowned medical centers in the world. Assuming there is a right decision (that one choice is better than the other), he could be choosing between life and death. It may not be as extreme as that, but without data on the two approaches, we can only speculate on the mortality and morbidity differences between the two. Here, we see one more instance where Peter's expertise in the medical field serves him well. It's highly likely the layperson hears what the Stanford physician says and is coerced under the weight of the institution's prestige. It is likely they are never even offered that third opinion. If they are, they are unlikely to elucidate the nuances between the two decisions. Having been in the position of *offering* these kinds of choices, Peter is well aware of what to consider.

It sounds like it should be relatively straightforward given his concerns. Peter doesn't want surgery, and now a specialist is telling him that not only is it unnecessary, but the time wasted on it can hurt him. Yet, Peter could not immediately agree. If surgery would drastically improve his chances for survival, then it would foolish to immediately dismiss the option. And so he discussed it further—first with Karen and his colleagues.

There was no consensus opinion.

"Go to MD Anderson. See what they want to do," one colleague told him. The sentiment was echoed. A local radiation oncologist, whom Peter trusted, told him he would be uncomfortable performing the recommended radiation in the malignant area of Peter's face. Such opinions only muddied the waters more.

During work, Karen was getting pulled aside by Peter's colleagues who wanted to use her as a mouthpiece for their opinion. "When physicians talk to me, they feel like they are talking to him, because they know I will relate everything to him. They also know I am here at work, and they know if they say something to me it will get to him," she remembers.

Peter had been undecided, but he was unhappy about the way this was unfolding. "I think [Peter] was unhappy with the lack of control..." Karen adds.

Finally, one of his close friends convinced Peter to do what, internally, he had wanted to the entire time. "Look, you go to MD Anderson, and you could be chasing this around forever," he told Peter. "You know that with or without surgery, you are going to need radiation and chemotherapy."

It was true. The more time Peter wasted, the worse his prognosis would be with any approach. That night, Peter and Karen had their final discussion on the matter.

"We decided—enough cutting, enough surgery. It set him back. Surgery you have anesthesia, you don't eat or drink, and at that point it was already difficult enough for him to do those things," Karen remembers.

"I said nothing doing. I felt that the whole surgery thing would kill me. I didn't think I would survive it...the complexity of it and the way I felt at the time. I was pretty beat up as it was, and I was still going to have to go through chemotherapy and radiation," Peter adds. "[The Stanford surgeon] called me and tried to convince me otherwise. He wasn't angry, but he thought it was in my best interests to do the surgery. He didn't have any outstanding arguments in pro, it was just his opinion. There wasn't any sound data or experience that he could promote as to why that would be so much better. I think 9 out of 10 times, a person off the street would have agreed to the surgery. My understanding of the medical community and medicine in general is much more than a layperson's."

Peter was set to begin chemotherapy and radiation. He thought he would have no problems with it. "I'm going to continue to work full time. I won't let it beat me down," he told the oncologist in his first meeting.

"It's going to be tough. The first three weeks are okay, but the last three weeks are going to be rough," the oncologist replied.

Peter pooh-poohed it. "Don't worry. I will be able to handle it."

The radiation therapy consists of daily treatments Monday to Friday for about six weeks. The chemotherapy was given once every three weeks for three times. Peter was being given a drug called Cis-Platinum, which has the potential side effect of kidney damage if not enough fluids are taken with its infusion. So Peter would have to stay at the chemotherapy clinic for several hours, to make sure he was well hydrated. It was vital that he continue that fluid intake for the next couple of days at home so that the Cis-Platinum could be flushed out of the body rapidly after it had done its job.

And for the first week Peter's premonition was right; he was absolutely fine. He would drive himself home from the chemotherapy center, and on the days when he wasn't getting infused, he would see patients in his clinic. Everything was going well.

One night on the following week Karen came home from work to find Peter sprawled on the couch, puking into a bag. He couldn't eat, couldn't drink, and was becoming severely dehydrated. Besides the obvious discomfort of dehydration, there was the danger posed by the Cis-platinum. Peter needed to stay well hydrated to avoid the kidney damage. Karen fetched some IV bags and needles from their office and set up an infusion at their house. The IVs quickly became a daily routine.

Peter continued to see patients as he swore he would, but it was increasingly difficult. His staff would triage the appointments, giving him updates on the patients so he could reduce the amount of time he had to spend in the rooms. In between seeing patients, he would lie down on the beds of the available rooms to take quick naps.

Why didn't he stop working?

"I always feel that when the going gets tough, the tough get going. I don't stop. It would have been nice. But I am a solo practitioner, and I don't have anyone to back me up. Most of my patients were too polite to ask; others were concerned," he explains.

Fair enough, but as a physician who had seen numerous chemotherapy patients, how did he not expect to be in this shape?

"I had been fit, a bodybuilder, in good shape, and ran every day…and yet I didn't feel very good. By the time I finished chemotherapy, I knew I was right. It really knocked the shit out of me. If I had that fourth surgery, I would have died. You know, I've been young and vigorous my entire life. Nothing much really bothers me, physically or mentally. And I've seen a lot of older people do this and then get back on with their life. And here I am young, and healthy. I was sixty-one when I started this. It is amazing how well it gets you."

Karen clarifies, "Ego, tough, male, doctor, he thought he would be fine. He thought it would be no big deal. He saw what it did to his patients, but I don't think he realized what it would do to himself since he was so much younger, and he was 240 pounds and he is always trying to lose weight and never could. He is a big guy and he is healthy, so I don't think he realized what the impact was going to be."

Peter could only keep up the tough façade he had been trying to project for so long. One evening, in the fourth week of chemotherapy, the oncologist received a phone call at home.

"It's kicking my ass…" Peter began.

An increasingly difficult problem was the issue of nutrition. Most IV solutions are meant only to supplement the actual volume of the body's fluid to keep blood pressure high and a person well hydrated. This is not the same thing as actually receiving real nutrition. And while you can also infuse that through the veins, it is seen more as a last resort because it is more ineffective than actually passing food through the intestines. Peter was not only feeling nauseated from the chemotherapy, but he also had inflammation from all the surgeries and now the radiation affecting his throat. It was incredibly painful for him to swallow. So even if the nausea was controlled, he couldn't eat. First, he was given liquid Lidocaine. Lidocaine is an anesthetic, so the idea was to coat the throat to block all the pain so he could eat something. This was not as effective as hoped.

So, if a patient can't eat, the next step is to get the food past the esophagus and go directly into stomach. This is where a nasogastric tube comes in. It's a long tube that is inserted directly into the nasal canal and pushed down the throat, through the esophagus, and into the stomach. It has multiple uses, one being that it can be used to help people like Peter get food down.

Now, if the idea of shoving a piece of tubing down the nose through the throat and into your abdomen sounds uncomfortable to you, you are not alone. Normally, a physician or nurse will insert the tubing for the patient by giving them sips of water to ease it through. Karen wanted to help Peter, but he shooed her away. He wanted to do it on his own.

In his bathroom, with a cup of water on the counter, Peter grabbed the tubing and measured out the distance he needed to insert. He did this by placing the tip at his nose and guessing how far along down it would be to his stomach and marking it on the tube. He lubricated the end with some gel, and with the mirror as his guide he pushed it into his nostril, grunting as he angled it downward. It tickled the back of his throat and he squeezed some water into his mouth. A spasm shook his sore throat, but the water helped him slide down the tube further. He took two strips of tape and wrapped the tube at the end of his nose. He grabbed some liquid food, sat down in his recliner, and squirted it through the tube.

Arduous, completely unnecessary, but pure Peter. He had gone from 245 pounds at the start of his surgeries to a tiny 180 pounds. And while the tube is uncomfortable while being inserted, it causes even more discomfort over time as it stays in place. While Peter had gotten it in without a sweat, after several days he couldn't take it anymore. He ripped it out and asked the oncologist for a PICC line (a type of IV access that is safe for home use). With his rapid weight loss and inability to eat, they had to start

TPN (total parental nutrition), which is just another way of saying they were feeding him through the vein instead of through the GI system. Intravenous nutrition is not sustainable over the long term, and if you think about it, going without eating would be incredibly disorienting, whether or not your body is receiving needed nutrients.

Peter still worked, despite Karen pleading with him not to. She called the oncologist. "You have to tell him to stay at home and rest; he doesn't listen to me," she told him.

The oncologist mulled it over and phoned Peter. "Peter, it may be a good idea to stay home and rest." They discussed how he had been holding up and the benefits of some time off from work. Surprisingly, Peter agreed.

"I think he realized, and he felt it, I think he just needed someone to you know, tell him that the world is going to go on. You need to take care of yourself right now. I think that had a huge impact on him. He still employed his staff, because he worries about his office, he worries about all that stuff," Karen explains.

"So he stopped working and dealt with being sick all the time with the chemo. We hooked up to the TPN at night; that way he wasn't connected to the IV pole all day. His body changed too. Besides the weight loss, he was cold all the time. Cold, cold, cold. Always cold. Stitches were cold. He worked out all the time, and lived in the country doing hard labor—but even his hands shrunk," she adds.

While Peter bemoaned the loss of his physicality, it was the loss of his drive that truly scared him and Karen. "It's like being poisoned. It is like you are dying. At one point, I really didn't care whether I died or not. It is like it took your vital energy, the spark of life stuff, and it goes away. Your vitality disappears," he explains.

Before Peter had gotten sick with the cancer, he was in a business-building mode. He had setup clinics in several towns of Central California including Lodi, Stockton, and Salinas. They had grown and expanded under his care, but with the drain on his vitality he simply couldn't keep it up. "He didn't want to do anything anymore. He just lost all the drive to work. He loves medicine, but he lost all that," Karen remarks.

Was he scared of death?

"No, not at all. It doesn't bother me. Partly because of my practice. I deal with death and dying all the time...part of [heart] disease is that it is a slow process that makes people slowly die, and I help them die with dignity. It is part of life. You can't have one without the other, unfortunately. It is also a conditioning thing. You get used to it. Rationalize it, I guess. [Karen] doesn't share the same attitude. She sees a lot of death too, but when it gets personal...she was pretty devastated by the whole thing," Peter remembers.

As brutal as the chemotherapy had been on him, it was only temporary. The real test would be the waiting period. If the cancer had not reappeared within five years, they could feel relatively assured that it would not return for good. This was based on statistics of mortality rates for people with peri-neural invasion from squamous cell carcinoma.

Eventually, Peter was able to eat food. Without the constant pounding of radiation, the inflammation in his throat reduced and he was able to swallow. Without the chemotherapy, he no longer felt nauseated. As time went on, he felt the old drive, the willpower to keep moving on to bigger and better things reigniting once again. It took almost a year to recover from the effects of chemotherapy, both physically and mentally.

Peter had changed though, that was for sure. Karen likes to tease him about becoming more sentimental. The two had been dating since 1995, and though they had lived with each other since 2000, the issue of marriage had never come up. Peter did not want to, and Karen had been through a divorce already and did not see the point. As Peter recuperated, he would joke with Karen, asking her where she would want to get married if they ever did.

When Karen asked why he posed that question, Peter responded dramatically, "Oh, maybe one day we'll *have* to get married." Then he dropped the subject.

Peter had also grown closer to his family during the sickness. He had been close to his brother beforehand, but with the reminder of his mortality he made an effort to see the rest of his family more often. Karen isn't sure if the sentimentality is from the cancer or just natural aging.

"Post-cancer, he cries a lot more at shows and TV. He has always been a sentimental guy. Now though he can hardly listen to a song, sad ones and happy ones, without getting tears in his eyes. TV shows, movies, where there are good storylines, with warm feeling stuff, he just get tears in his eyes," she laughs.

Peter has no comment.

In January 2008, a group of their friends put on a concert for them at their house. It had been a tradition of theirs every Christmas, for Peter and Karen to see them perform, but the past holidays Peter had been too sick to attend. After they finished their set, they all sat down in the living room. Peter threw out an innocuous question: "Would you be able to perform at our wedding?"

Karen's head whiplashed towards him. "I said what?!" she laughs.

Peter shrugged his shoulders. "We're getting married." He turned back to the band. "When can you sing at our wedding?" he continued. Ever the sentimentalist, Peter doesn't propose; he offers.

So with blessed simplicity they were married.

Peter awaits the end of his five-year sentence, maybe longer than that. In the meantime he sets out to retrieve what was taken from him. More than anything, he wants that vitality again.

What do we ultimately make of him, though? He's a proud man who feels comfortable controlling a situation. He isn't afraid of the prognosis, only the loss of control. And that's what is most at stake with our attempts at knowledge. We assume the more information we have, the more control we have. Is that true? Or are we only fooling ourselves? There's a difference between participating in our care, and perhaps being too proactive. Medical professionals dedicate years of their lives trying to master niches of the body; how can we possibly assimilate such knowledge in a practical manner spending one night perusing the web? On the other hand, it seems foolish to not educate ourselves on our own afflictions.

Peter had the misfortune of having too much knowledge and too little. He was calm, unperturbed by an initial diagnosis of squamous cell carcinoma that would frighten the average person. Yet, he had too little knowledge to know that he should have been desperate when he began having facial pain— because he was suddenly out of his element. Researching these diseases superficially only gives us the impression that we're in control. Perhaps it's best if we use what we read to ask more questions and seek answers. Perhaps it's best not to assume we know what's going on. Because sometimes even the experts don't.

The Other Way

ATLANTA, GEORGIA (1997)—JENNY was absent-mindedly rinsing dishes when it happened. Her eight-year-old son was in bed, fast asleep. Her boyfriend, a computer programmer, was watching television in the living room. As had happened so often in her life, she was about to undergo a radical experience. She loaded up another plate in the dishwasher and looked outside her window at the night sky. Under the soothing consonance of gurgling tap water, television color commentary, and insects chirping, she began to daydream.

Only, she found herself dreaming she was another person.

"I could see the ceiling of my son's bedroom. It was if I were looking at it from his point of view. All these questions began to race through my head. I felt very lost. I wouldn't say it was a vision. I'm not sure what to call it…a premonition maybe?" she remembers. She "regained consciousness" in front of the sink, which was threatening to overflow with water.

What did she do afterwards? Did she share her experience with her boyfriend?

She shrugs. "[He] would say weird crap like that doesn't happen."

Jenny would have a similar episode later on that year. Again, she felt she had been put in her son's place and was viewing the world from his eyes. Again, she felt the same feelings of fear, confusion, and loneliness. She wondered why she imagined her son feeling lost. What would cause him so much anxiety?

Let's put aside for a moment the nature of the vision (or dream or whatever you would like to call it) and focus on why it's important for Jenny. How she went into a trance, what she saw, when it happened, is trivial compared to the fact that she believes it happened. For people like Jenny, who are deeply spiritual, these are prophetic signs. Their spirituality is a personality paradigm that significantly shapes the way they act. To Jenny, these dreams indicated that her body (or soul) had an understanding beyond what she could comprehend. Inherently, it understood her future cancer better than anyone else.

Jenny is different. She is unafraid to admit what she likes, what she places importance in, even if it is not "normal." Walk into her home and you're hit by a whirlwind of household filigree. The walls are draped from corner to corner with arrowhead vine plants. The ceiling is a mural of the night sky, complete with constellations like Orion's Belt. The upper floor is covered with garden gnomes. It is different from the pervasive modern, sterile home décor. It gives you the feeling that this is a woman who marches to her own beat. It only makes sense she'd ignore standard protocol in her interactions with a healthcare system that is increasingly conformist. What was once considered an art by its practitioners is considered more and more to be a strict science that should adhere to a checklist method of action and evidence-based decisions. With the progress made in the field under such transformation, it is not hard to see why.

We began these sets of experiences with Mike's fight against small cell lung cancer, a battle that ultimately ended in his death three years later. From just a cursory glance at the statistics on cancer, it is not a surprising ending. It is also the reason no one handles the news of a cancer diagnosis with the same kind of apathy reserved for diseases from the flu to malaria, even though just fifty years ago malaria killed thousands in Europe and America. That's all fine and dandy, you're probably saying, but we've made great improvements in treating malaria. The total malaria fatality rate in the United States in 2007 was 1. We can actually cure and prevent it. You can't say the same thing about cancer, on the whole.

It is unfortunate the somber numbers on survival have tempered a view on how things have changed. Physicians around the world still have to do a verbal dance around the truth as they do their best to gently tell patients "there is no further active treatment available." So it is easy to forget or even ignore the progress made in fighting cancer. As dire as it is now, it's almost unimaginable to look at what it was like to have cancer even as recently as two decades ago.

From 1930 to 1990, breast cancer mortality changed very little. From 1990 to 2005 it decreased by 27%. Mortality decreased annually by 2.5% for white women and by 1.4% in black women. Of course, there is still work to do. In 2013 there were 110-121 new cases per 100,000 women and a mortality rate of 22 per 100,000 women in this country.

Things have improved significantly in the war on breast cancer due to a combination of events. With routine mammography, breast cancers are being detected earlier, leading to higher survival rates. Surgical techniques have evolved significantly; in fact you need look no further than the evolution of the mastectomy to see progress. In the early part of the 20th century, standard surgery used to be a radical mastectomy where the whole breast, lymph nodes in the underarm, and the chest muscle was removed. This surgery was developed by William Halsted, a European-trained surgeon at Johns Hopkins Medical Center. This was a disfiguring and debilitating surgery, as you can imagine, since almost half the torso was being removed—the logic apparently being that treatment for a crippling disease was to cripple the patient first.

Through the 1960s, 90% of the United States surgeons were performing what was called a Halsted mastectomy. In the 1970s a modified radical mastectomy was being done which was similar to the Halsted mastectomy, except the chest wall muscles were not removed. This was much less disfiguring and debilitating. In the early '80s, surgery evolved into lumpectomy (removal of the breast lump only and sparing most of the breast shape), removal of lymph nodes in the underarm, and radiation therapy. More recently, surgery has become more minimalist when possible, with lumpectomy and just sampling of the lymph nodes in the underarm along with radiation therapy. This has led to major improvement in patient's quality of life. Radiation therapy techniques have also improved, with much less collateral damage.

But more important has been the evolution of new medications for systemic treatment that include a number of new chemotherapy drugs, and numerous hormonal treatments as well as targeted treatments. One of the most important discoveries has been the finding of a target in the cancer cells itself, so treatment can be directed to the particular malignancy with much less collateral damage. HER-2/neu oncogene is a protein that lies in the cancerous cell and makes the cancer more aggressive. This is seen in 20% of women with breast cancer. Herceptin and other drugs related to Herceptin target this oncogene, thereby neutralizing it and help kill the cancer cell. This has been a major discovery in the treatment of breast cancer, leading to significant improvement in survival. A number of new medications targeting HER-2/neu oncogene have been recently approved by the FDA. So nowadays patients who are HER-2/neu oncogene positive, even if they have disease that has spread to the liver, bones, or elsewhere, can live a number of years with treatment.

So we're going to examine a breast cancer case that has elements of hope and disappointment. While Mike extended his life in spite of an unwavering terminal sentence, Jenny slowly slid toward an end that could have been preventable. She did it her way, but was it worth it?

If anyone can show how far cancer therapy has come along, it's Jenny. She hit rock bottom in her fight. Some of the blame lay in the healthcare system and some was due to her personal philosophy. "My kids would probably describe me as stubborn. My husband would probably describe me as a pain in the ass," she laughs.

The vast majority of her misery, though, is the work of an aggressive disease. Yet, she has been allowed to stumble and survive.

Therein lies the progress. There is room for error. *You're allowed to stumble now.*

Treatments have advanced to the point where they can pluck a person like Jenny away from what would have been certain death. Ironically, Jenny would not be described as one of Western medicine's staunch supporters. She's bucked against the system frequently, dedicated to remaining independent. It is a paradox that should be considered. For some reason, as medicine progresses, displeasure with and distrust of the health care field also seems to increase.

Jenny was born in Los Angeles, but lost her mother at a young age and was subsequently raised by her grandmother. When Jenny was eight years old, her grandmother, a Louisiana native, decided to move back to the South. This move wasn't permanent, and when Jenny was a teenager she moved back to California, only to later move back to the East Coast a decade later. That isn't exactly a pattern of stability, and you can see how it manifested itself in Jenny. She is tough and autonomous, both in nature and her beliefs. By 1997 she was living with her future husband and eight-year-old son in Atlanta. She was occupied as a registered nurse and worked with geriatric patients.

As is the case with most cancer patients, Jenny discovered her disease without those warning bell symptoms. One afternoon, after she came back home from work and was changing out of her work clothes, she noticed two lumps: one in each breast. Both felt different. The one on the left breast seemed rock hard, whereas the other felt tender.

"I would say the very first [thought] was disbelief. There was a lump there—it's wrong, but I also had an intuition that it was cancer. So it was a mix of stuff. And actually I guess my very first thought was my youngest son at the time was eight, and it was like I can't have this now because he is too young. It didn't fit. So that is what went through my mind then," she says. Despite her incredulity, Jenny's instincts were already gripping the truth. "I knew deep down it was [cancer]."

Breast cancer is often self-discovered. If the patient does not see the lump first, it is found by screening through mammograms. Although there is controversy surrounding the timing of mammograms, most organizations seem to agree that by the age of fifty, they are needed at least once every two years. The earlier the stage of breast cancer, the higher the cure rate, so screenings in general are absolutely helpful. If that is the case, though, why not just start screening at even younger ages? Part of the reason that mammograms are discouraged in young women is the breast tissue is not fatty enough at young ages. Fatty tissue makes it easier for the X-rays to pick up malignancies, so mammograms are much more accurate and useful in older women. Given the amount of false positives and low likelihood of actually finding a treatable disease, exposing younger women to radiation and errant procedures seems unnecessary.

Jenny saw a doctor who quickly arranged a biopsy. The results confirmed her intuition. One lump was cancerous, and the other was benign. The term lump and the term tumor are equivalent in this case.

But how could a tumor possibly be considered benign? In a tumor, one particular type of cell has escaped the normal constraints of growth and multiplied, forming a lump. The most important characteristic is the capacity to invade the surrounding tissue and the capability to spread elsewhere. If the tumor cells can invade and spread, they are termed cancerous or malignant; otherwise they are considered benign or noncancerous. So you can have lumps that aren't cancerous if they don't have the ability to invade further into the tissue and spread. Her doctor sat her down and explained what had to be done. Jenny would need surgery, followed by chemotherapy and radiation treatment. Most important though was the mastectomy, removal of her entire breast.

"You need an operation," her doctor told her.

"Well, I don't have a way to pay for it," Jenny replied. Although she worked as a nurse, it was on a per diem basis, so she had no insurance policy. "The biopsy alone had cost over $2000, so you can just imagine what the operation would be," Jenny says.

At the time of Jenny's diagnosis, Emory Hospital had two programs in place for those without insurance or the financial capability to pay for their treatment. Jenny was asked to speak with a social worker to determine her eligibility. In the meantime, she also needed a repeat mammogram in order to give the surgeons more information on her disease. Jenny made the earliest possible appointment at the busy Emory radiology clinic. It would be in a month. She figured that would buy enough time for the insurance issue to be settled. Frankly, she wasn't too concerned about moving along the process of her treatment as fast as possible.

What did scare her was delivering the news to her loved ones. Most daunting was explaining the situation to her eight-year-old son.

She finally settled on a direct approach.

"I have cancer," she told him.

"Is that bad or good?" he asked.

How could she possibly explain it to him?

"*Well, son, it's an abnormal proliferation of breast cells caused by sporadic and genetic mutations that eventually causes the body to break down*," would probably not work.

More importantly, how could she explain the possibility of her future death? "Years of playing Mario Bros. where the little guy dies and then comes back...I don't think he had any idea. At that age I didn't think I needed to explain it. So I just said I'm sick and I don't know if I'm going to get better or not," she remembers.

He handled it well, but did he really understand? It was impossible to tell.

It was easier for other family members. "My oldest son…there is a twelve-year difference [between my boys] and he was better able to handle it. He has helped me a lot. [He] is strong."

"When I first got the cancer, he was strong enough that I could say what I wanted to. He was somebody where I could say I'm dying and I want to talk about whatever, and he could accept it," she explains. Nothing was off-limits for their conversations, which was the way she wanted it. "He even got to the point where he was like—you know what, Mom? I want those gnomes [Jenny collects garden gnomes], so are you going to hurry up and die? We can joke about it."

Maybe that's unsettling to you, but Jenny finds comfort in bluntness. She doesn't want to dance around the truth, whether she is delivering it or it is being given to her. Uncertainty unsettles her.

That's why she was unusually anxious when the social workers had not gotten back to her after a month. They had gathered her information to help her qualify for financial aid. Without it, she wouldn't be in a position to receive the treatments.

Jenny went to her radiology appointment though she hadn't heard any news about the financial aid. As she sat in the waiting room at the radiology department, she thought about calling the social workers again. One month should have been enough time. Or was it? She wasn't sure how this was supposed to work. Maybe her anxiety was pressuring her? Was it possible things weren't actually moving that slowly? She was stressed so perhaps she wanted things to move faster than they could.

She looked around the sterile, bland room. She had been there an awfully long time. Or maybe she hadn't. She didn't have a watch on, there was no clock in the room, and she hadn't brought a magazine with her (she refused the office's compelling selection of *Arthritis Today* and *National Geographic* issues from the 1980s). *It was probably only five minutes and just feels like an hour. I'm anxious and it feels longer than it is,* she thought.

A few more minutes went by. She paced back and forth, then began to reason it out. *This is a big clinic, very busy, so it should take a long time*, she thought.

A few more minutes passed. *This is ridiculous.*

She opened up the door and looked down the dark hallway. That's not literary dramatics; the lights were literally turned off. The other rooms were open, empty, and also unlit. The busy clinic was absolutely silent. Jenny picked up her purse and walked outside. She could hear the faint "tick tacks" of keyboard typing. She entered the main lobby. The secretary was by herself, finishing up last-minute scheduling. Jenny looked at the clock. It was nighttime. The office was closed. She hadn't been waiting for minutes—it had been *hours.* The doctor had left a while ago. He had either forgotten she was in the room or hadn't even known at all. The secretary was also surprised to see her; she had no idea that somebody had been left behind in a room.

As the secretary fished the key out of her pockets to open the exit, Jenny thought again about the lack of news from the social workers.

Maybe one month was a long time.

"I was just disappointed by the way it was all happening," she remarks.

She received her mammogram the next day and was told to wait for the surgeons to call her.

As far as the social workers, though, she would not receive news from them until three months later. When they finally did call, they told Jenny she had been denied.

"Okay, which program?" Jenny asked, figuring that she would at least qualify for one of them.

"I dunno, it just says you were denied," the social worker responded. Jenny persisted, insisting she was being screened for two programs. The worker hung up after promising to get back to Jenny.

Several weeks later, Jenny received another phone call from the office. It was a different social worker on the line this time. "Ma'am, you've been denied the program," the somber worker told her.

Jenny sighed. "I know this already! Which one is it?"

There was silence on the other line.

"I'll get back to you," the other person finally replied.

When she did, Jenny found out she had been denied both programs. Among the reasons offered for the denial was Jenny's hourly wage exceeded the minimum by one dollar. Immediately after the explanation from the social workers, she received a phone call from the surgical offices at Emory. The staffer was reviewing Jenny's file, and wondered why Jenny had refused to talk to the doctor about reconstruction surgery. "I didn't refuse to talk to the doctor. I've been waiting for [you] to call me!" Jenny snapped.

It was silent on the other line, until the staffer chuckled. "Oh, the computer chip in my head isn't working. This says referral, not refused."

Jenny grew irate as she listened. "I had been waiting for—" Jenny pauses. "Everything just wasn't working right, okay? So um, in the meantime I was trying alternative medicines."

If we consider Jenny's background and personality, this should come as no surprise. Should she surrender herself to the doctors in the shadows, the bumbling nurses, and the clueless office staff? No way.

Alternative medicine is different and unknown—seductive adjectives for Jenny. Most tempting of all is it demands Jenny be proactive. She's the one searching for the treatments, buying them, learning about new methods, exposing herself to options that most people would never consider. Though limited, *she* is in control. It's medicine as an *art.* So there's Jenny, heeding the manifesto of a system that so far had fumbled her care as her own sickness flourished. And when she tries alternative therapy? She marches to the beat of her own drum.

So what is alternative medicine? It is any means of healing or treatment that does not fall within the realm of conventional Western medicine. It is based on cultural, historical, or social traditions. Its critics usually claim, not without merit, that most alternative medicine is not backed by evidence. That wasn't a concern to Jenny, though; she jumped at every possible treatment she could get her hands on.

"There was Essiac tea. Most of them I found on the web, through books, stuff like that. I got the Essiac tea through health food stores. The person who invented it was a nurse and years ago she had good results with it in patients who had cancer."

"I tried acupuncture, I have oriental things… it's cool. Mushrooms and lizards and everything and you make a tea out of it and I can really feel a difference. There is this drug that is illegal from Germany. I tried some of that," Jenny continues.

"Were there any benefits to these treatments?" I ask her.

Jenny pauses before replying. "I felt that it was helping. I would feel better. Some more than others. Some were strange. I got these heavy waters; supposedly if your body is very alkaline you won't have cancer. So I took caesium and potassium water. I have a book by some doctor who is practicing in Mexico, because apparently a lot of what they do is illegal here. She even made this machine that runs on a battery and works on the same principle as acupuncture—I've tried all different things. None are a cure, but I think they are all of some benefit."

This latter treatment was the invention of Dr. Hulda Clark, a controversial alternative medicine practitioner who believed the root cause of every disease was a parasite, the intestinal fluke. This was described in her book *The Cure for All Diseases*. She claimed all human disease was related to a parasitic infection. She also claimed to cure all disease, including cancer and HIV/AIDS. She claimed to destroy these parasites by "zapping" them with electrical devices that she marketed. These machines were illegal in the United States because the US Federal trade commission and Food and Drug Administration found these claims to be "bizarre," scientifically unfounded, and fraudulent. Dr. Clark died in 2009 from myeloma (a type of blood cancer).

The benefits are indefinable. Jenny's feelings are not tangible markers that can be compared patient to patient. You might wonder what's so bad about that. Some critics would point out this can all be a placebo, but that really isn't a problem. Much of modern medicine also has placebo effects. As long as the patient feels better, isn't that really enough? We've talked about improving the quality of life as one of the two major goals in healthcare, so if a person is feeling better, hasn't their quality of life improved? Furthermore, there hasn't been any evidence that any of these treatments actually harm anyone. Mushroom and lizard tea sounds disgusting (can't sugarcoat that one) but it never hurt Jenny's cancer. We'll ignore the financial implications of being swindled, because cost unfortunately is a shared flaw with Western medicine, and see how Jenny's enthusiasm toward alternative medicine affected her future.

In the meantime, Jenny felt as though she was affecting her care. And when it came to Dr. Clark's medicine, it is easy to see why she was so enthusiastic.

Dr. Clark's claims are different from conventional medical treatments in one big way: they claim to *cure*, not *treat*. That's an attractive claim for people frustrated with the treatment of cancers. In many cases, those with advanced cancer are told to forget about the idea of a cure. How is it possible, with all the money we've poured into cancer research, we haven't come up with a cure? Is it possible the country is not doing enough to fight cancer?

The War on Cancer was declared by the United States Government when President Richard Nixon signed the National Cancer Act of 1971. This legislation was designed to dramatically increase research efforts. At the signing of the bill, President Nixon said, "I hope in the years ahead we will look back on this action today as the most significant action taken during my administration."

According to Vincent DeVita, director of the National Cancer Institute (NCI) from1980 to 1988, "the incidence of cancer in the United States started dropping in 1990 and has continued to drop every year since, and so has mortality. And the morbidity from cancer comparing 1971 to 2005, is like night and day.... So, every benchmark of the mandate has been hit." But even with the dramatic improvements made, most of the common cancers (lung, colon, breast, pancreas) remain incurable if discovered at an advanced stage.

We are getting better at treating cancer, but the cure rate for advanced cancer is still nothing to boast about. With futility in fighting a disease, it is easier for people to accept the lack of a cure. But when the layman sees a healthcare field that seems to be infinitely focused on propping patients up from the brink of death with harsh treatments, it becomes a breeding ground for skepticism. Whereas people would have turned to alternative medicine out of desperation, we now get patients like Jenny who resort to it out of frustration with the current system. She didn't want to be tethered to medicine for the rest of her life. The promises that alternative medicine made were enough to lure her to it.

As bizarre as it is, the fact that medicine has become less of an art and more of a strict science has a lot to do with this. Picture the doctor of the last century, a man/woman who is seen as the gatekeeper between life and death. They are revered. Today, they are cogs in a system that has to function in certain ways that have been predefined. The mysticism of the cure has been replaced with the certainty of evidence-based treatment. Perhaps that's why there is less trust in the healthcare field these days. It's a business now. The mom and pop stores might inspire greater trust and better relationships, but arguably they don't operate as efficiently as the megastores. Healthcare has advanced under the same principle. We have better results. People are living longer. And yet there are folks like Jenny, whose alternative medicines are not slowing the progression of her disease, offer no concrete evidence of improvement either in symptoms or lifespan, and yet they feel more positive about those treatments than they do about the rigorously studied triad of chemotherapy, radiation, and surgery. You can't even claim that Jenny's knowledge is pure ignorance; she had worked as a nurse for years in a Western healthcare system and was certainly well versed in allopathic medicine.

Although Jenny had dipped her toe into the waters of alternative medicine, she had not ignored conventional therapy. There was the payment issue. She was not wealthy enough to afford her treatments directly, and at the same time her wages were high enough to disqualify her for government aid. She had only one option left to finance payments for her treatment: marriage. Her boyfriend at the time wanted to get married. Jenny had already been divorced twice and did not see the point of marrying again. However, if she did get married she could be placed under the umbrella of her new husband's health insurance plan. Jenny had refused so far, not wanting to walk down the aisle again.

And so her cancer progressed, steadily eroding more and more of her breast.

While she insisted her alternative treatments were helping, the most that they could achieve was alleviation of her symptoms. The cancer had grown to the point where it severely distorted her breast tissue. Jenny was determined to keep anyone at her work from knowing about the situation. "I didn't want anyone to know that I have cancer. I was just like 'Can I have more hours?' Because there are a lot of people that I haven't told. I'm just strange that way. Even now I haven't told [them]. I have some distant family that I keep in touch with in Louisiana…it would just make them sad. I've always been the strong one. Some people can't handle it. It would just make them sad. So it's like why tell them? You know? They would always be calling me and aggravating me and making me do stuff," she explains.

"It is more like, I feel that it would hurt their feelings and it would be a bother, so why do it? It is distant relatives, so it's like Christmas cards, phone call twice a year. I have a girlfriend and I didn't tell her for six or seven years. She moved away, so it was like why bother her? She called me and said, 'I haven't seen you in a while so I'm coming to visit.' So I figured it's about time to tell her. She cried. She is not a strong person. A good friend, but not a strong person."

Early on, the most she had to do was simply not tell other people. When the cancer eroded the surface of her breast and began to bleed, it became more difficult to hide.

"I first started feeling pain—it was like a cut, like if you had a stab wound or something. I didn't do much with the pain. It was more like you had an open cut. It was bleeding and more or less rotting, pieces of my flesh turned orange and crispy and fell off. It was kind of a disgusting," she remembers. Cancer by itself is not painful. Pain is usually caused by the cancerous cells infiltrating nerve endings or bone or any other tissue that has a lot of nerve endings. This is why most cancer, like a tumor lump found in the breast, is not painful. Jenny began having pain because the cancer was invading tissue.

Having blood on your work uniform is an obvious way to invite questions. So Jenny woke up early every morning to wrap the open tissue sores with gauze. Days, then weeks, then months went by and no one knew. But every day the wound grew bigger. It bled more. And more gauze was needed to pad it. At some point, someone was going to notice that Jenny was taping an entire blanket on her chest.

Jenny stayed the course, though, until she finally reached a point she could no longer ignore. It had been a normal day. Jenny had come back from an exhausting day of work. She was ready to relax under a hot shower. In the bathroom, she took her bra off. She heard a small rattle, as if something had fallen onto the floor. She instinctively reached to her ears, thinking that an earring had fallen, but both earrings were in place. She looked down. She saw what looked like a piece of pink-orange flesh. She looked down at her breast. It looked different. She pressed on it with her finger and suddenly her entire nipple fell into her hand.

Although uncommon, this is certainly possible. Remember, the cancer had been growing. It had invaded into the surrounding tissues, causing pain and also destruction. It had interfered with the blood supply to the breast tissue. When that happens, areas that are completely cut off from blood will die. And dead tissue can come right off.

That was the week her boyfriend had planned a trip to New York for a weekend work conference. Jenny, in panic mode, went along with him. A Daoist temple in the city was going to be her last ditch effort. There, she explained her situation. The stunned Daoists were blunt with her.

"There is nothing we can do," they told her.

Any treatments they had, she already used. She needed chemotherapy, radiation, and surgery. She needed health insurance to pay for it. Jenny made her decision right then and there.

She called up her boyfriend to tell him the good news.

The wedding he had been asking for was about to occur that day.

"Find two rings and come meet us," she told him over the phone. The temple's own Daoist priest was going to marry them. Jenny's happy memories: "And it was cool how everything happened, because everyone at the meditation center was invited to the wedding. Some people had a car and went shopping and got a dress, one of the girls went and picked wildflowers, I had a bouquet and people had drums, and sang and I had a wedding." Yes, Jenny was quite the hipster.

She had been diagnosed in 1997. She was married in 1999. Two full years had gone by without the treatments she needed. Think about that interval. In most every other story, people panicked if they couldn't get the wheels in motion within a week. Jenny had to live with the burden of disease for two years!

When she had first been diagnosed, she was told she needed surgery first and then she would undergo chemotherapy and radiation. That treatment plan would have to be changed. Remember, with surgery you can take out only so much of the flesh. Doctors wouldn't remove half her torso just to get rid of a cancer. Although technically feasible, it can lead to significant deformities, higher incidence of infections, delayed healing, requirement of skin grafts, and other issues. So then the option of tumor shrinkage prior to surgery becomes critically important. The smaller it is, the more easily it can be surgically removed. This was done in Jenny's case. She would receive chemotherapy for several months and then be re-evaluated for surgery.

"Just thinking back on the whole thing, screw the insurance—it was a little lump at the time…I [just] didn't know how I would have gotten the money because she quoted me the costs and it was way expensive," Jenny laments.

Her procrastination had landed her in the chemotherapy clinic prior to surgery.

"My first experience with chemo was actually scary. Here is the thing that bothered me. I knew what chemo was and how your hair falls out and…yeah. So they bring me into this room, I felt like I was a cow being herded into something. There were thirty people in there, all with IVs. The first thing, I guess being a nurse, I was like what is with the confidentiality. Everybody knows everything, everyone knows everyone's drug bag, the thing I was almost in shock, all I am is a number and there is no confidentiality. I felt that I didn't need to share that I had cancer with everyone else and here is this whole crowd of people. I just wanted to be in a room all by myself. That is what I pictured, not knowing how they did this."

Yes, Jenny is a number. Western medicine is conformist. It has to be. If you want to collect evidence on treatments, they have to be standardized. Everything needs to be the same. Patients like Jenny have to be a ticker in the system. There is no other way for it to work.

Jenny wanted to stay hidden. "But there's no way it isn't discussed in front of everyone—you hear how much people weigh... the bowel things...I just wanted to crawl away and hide. You just get used to it," she says.

"I mostly kept to myself. After a while I got used to it, and if people would say something, you'd start talking to them. It is like there is no way anyone can really write about it or prepare you in a book [not helping me here, Jenny]. They can tell you your hair falls out....You see all these people throwing up. Some in the clinic, some all over the place...I would just lay there. I couldn't eat. I was just totally miserable. You can't explain it. It is not like this hurts, and that hurts. It's not a hurt. It is like if you felt nauseous, but all of you felt nauseous...your legs, arms, just miserable. You can't say it is a pain, but everything is uncomfortable, everything is extremely uncomfortable."

Unlike other patients, Jenny hated to rely on other people for her treatment. If the treatment finished, she would give the busy nurses a few minutes before she decided to relieve them of their duties by taking the IV out herself. She was asked not to do that, but it really didn't matter to Jenny. The nurses could only laugh as they saw the looks on other patients' faces as Jenny pulled out her own IV.

Jenny didn't care. She was doing it her way.

Beyond the pain, there was something else that bothered her—aesthetics.

"The other part was that I aged like fifteen years in one year. I used to be nice to look at, but I got old and ugly instantly. I've gone through the hair falling off three times, but it's like your skin gets a different texture. First of all you feel like everything—your skin is different, it's not even you anymore, it gets old and wrinkly. Also like your eyelashes and eyebrows fall out, and mine have never grown in. My hair has grown back but not those. But yeah, it doesn't happen overnight, but you can see it—like over fifteen years in terms of looks in over a year," she explains.

She continued, "It hurts when your hair falls out. You can comb your hair and clumps fall out. They said to shave your hair first, but I didn't because a couple of the people at the clinic said they had really thick hair and by the time their sessions ended they still had a little hair left. So I was like, well maybe I'll also have some hair left. It wouldn't hurt, but it was uncomfortable, you could feel it coming out." In the end she lost all her hair and relied on a fishing hat to cover her head.

Jenny had switched jobs at this point. She was no longer working in the geriatrics department, but rather with troubled youth. "By this time, I was working with children. It was abused children with behavioral problems. It was like an outdoor facility, so I was working there at the time, when I was getting chemotherapy.

They had different group settings, like they had one whole clinic which was just for sex offenders and murderers who were children. They had different age groups, and um, these were really severe behavioral problems and the reason was that most of them were abused. I was the nurse and I gave them the drugs, I was with them there for everything, I would do everything with them. For fifteen kids they had one nurse and five counselors to watch them. Basically you were mother and gave them meds."

Jenny was still in the habit of hiding her ailment. She didn't want to invite questions and comments, especially not with the new people in her work life. Hiding a lump, even a bleeding one, is a lot easier than hiding the effects of chemotherapy, though.

"One of the things was…it was really difficult once my hair fell out. If they found out, these kids would use anything, because of their behavioral problems. Once my hair fell out, I had a wig, and I was like, I hope these kids don't find out it's a wig, otherwise it will be in the toilet."

I've painted a picture of a very strong-willed woman at this point, but I think it would be unfair to not show some of Jenny's fears. It seems she wanted to be left alone, but it feels more like she was afraid to burden those around her. Jenny was so committed to independence that she had difficulty maintaining connections even with those closest to her.

"At times I would feel awful, laying in bed, and would tell my husband to call the doctor and what to say to the doctor. And for whatever reason, he couldn't do it. So I was like okay, if I am going to do this I can't rely on anybody. He couldn't say no or authority bothers him or whatever. Okay, so it was showing me that I couldn't depend on anyone but myself."

It seems extreme, but Jenny was preparing herself. She wanted to be mentally ready for the toughest moments in life, and she felt that self-reliance was the only way she could reach it. "Someday I'm not going to get another chance," she tells me. "And I'm going to be laying there by myself dying. I think our culture is afraid of death and no one wants to acknowledge it."

"It's almost as if you throw them into a tank of snakes and they're afraid of snakes. That first night they're going to be like oh my god, all these snakes. But they can't stay at that pitch forever. After a while, you wonder what's next? At first you are like, why me? Then soon you go into why me, what am I to learn from this? Then you go into okay, I have it, what's next...."

What you notice with Jenny is the irreverence she has for the system and society's norms. There is good and bad to that. One advantage is she obviously lacks the generous amount of fear that permeates the rest of the population. The disadvantage is there is a lot to revere about the power of medicine. To make the ill feel better, to deliver relief in times of pain—these are not measures that came about easily and without struggle. To dismiss them so easily means you also don't realize how lucky you are to live in an era when there are so many treatment options available. Much of the public may distrust modern medicine, but that doesn't mean it is the right thing to do. Sometimes it causes us to leave options on the table that we should be picking up.

Jenny's irreverence reared its head when eight months after she began chemotherapy, she decided she wanted to move to California. The doctors had already begun to plan her surgery, but Jenny was still stinging from the scolding she received when she first started treatment. "The doctor had told me that I had two years even if I followed everything they recommended," she remembers, still smarting from the criticism of starting medical treatment too late.

"I was just like, screw it. I'm going to California. If I'm going to die, I'm going home to die…always wanted to go back to California," she says. She told her husband she was moving back home.

"I can't a get job there. And I'm from New York. I'm not moving anyplace where the earth moves," he told her.

"Okay, I'll move by myself," Jenny replied.

Stuck between a rock and Jenny, he reluctantly decided to put an application online and see if he would get any offers. Within twenty-four hours he had eighty-seven hits, and most doubled his salary.

Jenny was headed home. She didn't care that she had stopped her treatments on a dime.

There's good and bad to irreverence. Jenny was going to pay for hers. Let's fast forward to the next stage of Jenny's treatment.

"With all the different screw-ups, I was getting a message that this doctor and clinic [wasn't] for me. So we [moved] and I went to see a doctor in Castro Valley [in Northern California], and she looked at me and said, I don't want to rush you but if you don't have this done within a week you are really pushing it, because you should have had this done a year ago. The doctor in California was the complete opposite [of her Atlanta physicians]. Zipiddidy doo dah. Scheduled it immediately and made me really feel like I was supposed to be there. So I had the operation; they did a radical mastectomy. She said it was in 60% of my lymph nodes. And then after that I had radiation on the site."

According to the follow-up scans, Jenny appeared to be in remission. Let's think about how extraordinary this is. Despite the lack of an absolute cure for breast cancer, she was still able to fight back the disease even after it had been allowed to grow unhindered for two full years.

Jenny had been knocking on death's door, and she wanted a change from her work at the hospital and youth development groups. She took up a job at hospice. Part of this was cathartic. Although Jenny had no urge to impart her cancer stories to others, especially those who were suffering, she felt as though her own experience had proven her strength. She could be a rock to those who were approaching the end.

"How did you approach that?" I asked her.

She paused, clearly bothered by what she was about to tell me. "I had to be a really hard person. For example, I have one patient who died of cancer who was thirty-one and she had an eighteen-month old baby and the husband just lost it—he actually forgot he had the baby. He was so upset with his wife dying. So I had to be the strong one in all of this. I had to…talk to him." She explained to the patient that death was a part of life. She wanted him to be strong for his child. Even for someone as tough as she was, it had to be a difficult conversation.

"I wanted to go someplace else and cry," Jenny adds. "But I couldn't, because that would just make it worse for the family."

Jenny shared another story. "I didn't let the fear overtake me, whereas other people just crumble and give up. Another example, a patient in hospice…when I first got [her] she was 5'7" and weighed sixty-five pounds. That was when I had her at her heaviest—she died shortly after, weighing about fifty pounds. Her condition was really bad and she was living in a house with no electricity. She was going to be evicted except they didn't want to throw out this terminally ill patient in the end stages and she looked at me and said, 'I don't know what to do: should I fight it or not? If I fight it, I don't know where I am going to live or where I am going to go.' She was like, it is probably better not to fight. Her living conditions were in such bad shape that she gave into it and died a few weeks later. What I am saying is you need to have a strong will, you need to try other things whether they work or not."

I spent an earlier chapter (Marty) detailing why it was okay for a patient's attitude to deviate from the norm, simply because the right attitude for any patient is what is comfortable for them. It is no different with Jenny. While I might disagree with the idea that fear causes a person to succumb (the poor lady who was about to be evicted was in a rotten of a situation), it is a vital concept to Jenny. Attitude is the only thing that could have propelled her to live with a cancer without the benefit of treatment for over two years. In her mind, it was a near miracle for her to still be alive—a miracle that came into fruition from a stew of the supernatural (her dogmatic belief in alternative medicine) and the depths of the human spirit to persevere in intolerable situations. At the end of the day, Jenny has to be comfortable with who she is. She has to rationalize her actions, their consequences, and she exports the belief onto those around her. She is uncomfortable with the idea of weakness because it doesn't work in her story.

"Do you think people succumb faster if the attitude is not there?" I ask her.

"Yes," she responds. "I also think cancer is almost like…it's my belief that everything is for a reason. Just sitting around in the chemo, it seems everyone has had some major trauma or something they experienced in their life like maybe six months to a year before they had cancer. So I think it may be related in some way to—they don't know what causes the cells to mutate in some way. My own theory is that some major stress causes it to mutate…[stress] may be a trigger."

"You are saying it is not a good idea to crumble, but at the same time it seems like it would be hard for someone who isn't tough to do so?" I counter.

"You go through stages…Kubler-Ross stages," Jenny responds. "She has different stages of death and dying, it depends on some people who get cancer, but if they more or less tell you it is a death sentence, go through the stages and try to get to the end. Everyone will die and you have an opportunity to open your eyes and be more aware of it. Personally, I think the reason I am still here despite doctors telling me that I might not be here now is that I have learned from it, and there is no reason for me to die from it anymore."

For those of you wondering, Elisabeth Kubler-Ross defined a model of the stages of grief that was introduced in 1969. It describes five discrete stages of the process by which one copes with grief and tragedy, especially after a terminal diagnosis. The stages all popularly known by the acronym DABDA, include denial, anger, bargaining, depression, and acceptance.

After the surgery, Jenny had been doing well, but there is no guideline for how long treatments should be continued for breast cancer.

She bounced from clinic to clinic, looking for an oncologist that suited her needs. Most physicians she spoke to were uncomfortable with her approach to treatment. Jenny was not enthusiastic about continuous medical therapy, and wanted to use it in only the direst of circumstances.

Earlier, I mentioned what a miraculous feat it was to be able to save someone from the brink of death. Yet, there are limits.

With a disease of progression, there has to be constant vigilance in order to stay alive. Without a cure, one can't just step away from the responsibility of taking care. However, this is tiring. It drains a person's energy and finances.

You can imagine how Jenny, who obviously did not like the burden of being tethered to someone or something (such as medication) and had concerns over her finances was not placed in a good situation.

She met the final oncologist of her life in October 2007 after switching from physician to physician in the past few years. She wanted someone who wouldn't force her into compliance. At that time she was on was on Letrozole, Herceptin, and Aredia. Letrozole is an anti-estrogen hormone given in pill form. Herceptin is the targeted treatment without the usual side effects of chemotherapy. Aredia is a drug that helps in bone repair and decreases further bone destruction of any cancer that invades the bones.

Jenny had responded remarkably well to these treatments. Her quality of life was not only improving, but good. The one issue that persisted was swelling of the abdomen. It's a condition called malignant ascites (fluid) and it is caused by fluid production from cancer cells in the abdomen. However, a CT of her chest, abdomen, and pelvis in November 2007 showed even the ascites was decreased and the nodules of her liver metastases were shrinking.

Six months later, her oncologist wanted to repeat the CT to confirm continued efficacy of the drugs she was still using. Jenny refused. The oncologist was puzzled, but he had come to expect Jenny's mercurial approach to her care.

"This is the only way for me to pick up early disease if you have a recurrence. It lets us know if the treatment needs to be changed," he explained.

She shook her head. "I know my body, and if the disease progresses I will be aware of it." Her physician knew she wouldn't budge, so he dropped the subject.

The treatments continued for another year, again without any changes. Jenny still refused to get imaging. Finally, in July of 2009 she changed her mind and agreed to get a CT of the chest and abdomen as well as an MRI of the brain.

Everything came back normal. Her blood tests showed no abnormalities. Profiles of her heart function were great. A year later, Jenny asked to stop all intravenous treatment. She wanted to stop the Herceptin for three months, quit the Aredia, but continued Letrozole, which was an oral medication. Despite the fact she was feeling well, she really needed to continue these treatments; they were critical to her survival. The oncologist had reluctantly agreed to all the changes, mainly because he knew and understood Jenny's behavior based on her history of moving from doctor to doctor. It would be hard getting her to resume IV treatments even if she needed it. His suspicion was confirmed when three months later she asked to not resume Herceptin.

"Without Herceptin, there is good chance the disease would grow back in the near future," he explained. It didn't matter. Jenny wanted to be free.

I asked her oncologist, "Why did you agree to stopping her treatment?"

"Well, by this time I knew Jenny very well and I knew she would do what she wanted to do, so trying to force her to do things would not work. I did explain to her the danger of stopping treatment in great detail, not once but repeatedly, but her mind was made up. Besides, my job is to give information and knowledge to patients, not to force them to make decisions which I think are correct, and also it is not my job to pass judgment on their behavior and their paradigm of thinking."

December 2011 – The oncologist received a call from Jenny. She was having headaches and was unsteady on her feet. She was finding it difficult to maintain her balance.

She readily acquiesced to an MRI of her brain. The scan showed multiple lumps in her brain consistent with spread of her breast cancer to the brain.

"I started her on dexamethasone, which is a pill to decrease pressure in the brain, and also referred her for radiation therapy. She became very weak after the radiation therapy, but her headaches decreased and her unsteadiness improved. This was very typical of Jenny—as long as she was feeling well she did not want significant active treatment. Unfortunately, by the time she agreed to treatment it was too late," the oncologist remembers.

By February 2012 Jenny was having difficulty breathing. She was admitted to the hospital. X-rays showed evidence of fluid in the lungs on both the right side and left side. She had the fluid drained from the lungs, which improved her breathing. But she was clearly deteriorating. The oncologist asked her to restart treatment, but she refused.

Jenny died on March 6th, 2012.

I apologize if you were expecting a happier ending, if Jenny's death came more suddenly than you expected, but that's the nature of cancer. The human body has surprising ranges of resiliency and vulnerability. So despite everything she was able to endure, at some point it became too much.

Jenny had Stage IV breast cancer that was estrogen receptor positive and HER-2/neu oncogene positive. These patients can respond and keep the cancer at bay with a combination of Herceptin given intravenously every three weeks and an anti-estrogen pill. This combination is well tolerated with very reasonable side effects. Both of these medications are not chemotherapy and do not have cause nausea, vomiting, hair loss, and low blood counts that are commonly seen with most chemotherapeutic treatments. The present recommendation is to continue Herceptin for as long as possible, as long as the patient is responding to treatment. Jenny was also getting Aredia, which helps with controlling pain in the bones, and helps repair bones damaged by cancer. She had evidence of spread of cancer to the bones as well, so continuing on Aredia was also important for her. Unfortunately, Jenny's refusal to continue the treatment caused her rapid decline and ultimately her demise. She could never reconcile her desire for independence and control with the treatment for her condition.

"She was with me for five years and told me that this was longest she had stuck with any physician, mainly because I listened to her and she felt that she was participating in the decision-making process. She felt she was in control. Unfortunately she made multiple wrong and ultimately lethal decisions. Had she followed the usual and accepted treatment recommendations, there is a good chance that Jenny would have been alive and in good shape at this point in time," the oncologist laments.

I don't want this to seem as if I'm picking on Jenny. She was a very strong woman whom I respected. She had her own goals and probably achieved them. But it would be wrong for me to not point out that she decreased her own chance for survival. Jenny understood the risks, was medically educated, and was fine accepting it. Her decisions and how they affected her, family, and friends could only truly be calculated by her. So I can't fault her decisions. But there are plenty of people who make uninformed decisions about their treatment plans. They're sold on quackery, on claims that are too good to be true. But we want to believe those claims. We want to believe that somewhere out there is a hidden cure and we can find it. It's a glimmer of hope in this terrifying fight.

Just as important though, is that we not delude ourselves. Jenny had strong, *strong*, views on life and death. She knew she had to. Even if she tried alternative medicine, she understood what she was in for. Lizard tea and electrolyte batteries weren't salvation; they were tools to help her keep fighting. She needed all the help she could get. She knew that sometimes doing it your way hurts.

The Age-Old Question

CANCER IS NOT a hopeless condition. It is formidable and deadly, but society has made great strides in fighting it. We expect only progress in the future. But there is another factor that often complicates the condition of cancer patients, and it is a terminal process for which there is no cure: age. The two are naturally intertwined. Cancer is an inherent mechanism of the body normally controlled by our immune system, but sooner or later the natural fail-safes of the body falter. Given enough time, anybody can be afflicted with a cancer. As the average lifespan continues to climb, the incidence of malignancy will only go up. The average age of the cancer patient will also increase. Cancer is primarily a disease of older people, with incidence rates increasing with age for most cancers. More than 60% of cancers are diagnosed in people age sixty-five and over.

With the harsh effects of chemotherapy, radiation, and surgery, there are dilemmas about using aggressive treatments on the elderly. There are financial implications as well. In an increasingly resource-constrained world, more focus is placed on what exactly constitutes a "necessary" treatment. This isn't constrained to the world of oncology. Elderly patients have the lion's share of comorbidities and subsequently health care costs. How we approach this is going to be controversial. This discussion won't be easy or neat. Note the hysteria around "death panels" during the "Obamacare" legislation in 2009 and you can see how frenzied the discussion can be. Are there future patients just waiting to be financial casualties? Should a person in their 70s, 80s, or 90s even be considered for a measure as aggressive as chemotherapy?

Who should have the right to decide which treatment modalities should be employed? And how do we decide which options are reasonable? These are important questions, and to delve into them we are going to look at two senior citizens who were faced with these same dilemmas. They took different approaches to their cancer diagnosis and treatment. Their outlook and treatment decisions stemmed from their pasts in World War II and also the numerous players surrounding them (family, friends, physicians, and the medical system) who each had their own motives. When you look at the factors that affect elderly care, it becomes clear that financial repercussions alone would be a very poor way to address the issue.

Gunther was born in Pomerania, a former region in Germany annexed to Poland following World War II. In December 1942, five months shy of his eighteenth birthday, he was drafted into the German Army, which was mandatory at the time, regardless of work or study. He was part of an elite division, used initially to greet dignitaries, but with the advent of World War II his unit was soon transferred to the front lines. As they were well supplied, they became the "fire department" division that was plugged into particularly weak areas for the German front lines.

After the war, with the help of a family friend, he and his wife Erica were sponsored so they could immigrate to the United

States. They've lived here ever since. Gunther has gone from being a soldier to a police commissioner in Germany to manager of a car dealership in California. Though he and Erica never had children, they've enjoyed life thoroughly. In 2009, at the age of eighty-four, Gunther was diagnosed with breast cancer. As with every patient, he was told that some combination of surgery, radiation, and chemotherapy was necessary in order for him to have a better chance of survival. On paper, with Gunther's age and lack of family, it would seem reasonable for him to forgo any aggressive treatment. Some might even argue he should be denied treatment. Even if the procedures salvaged him from cancer, as an octogenarian his chance of dying from another condition every year is high. The average life expectancy of an eighty-year old is seven years. Without cancer, the "average" Gunther would live only three more years at the time of diagnosis. But Gunther immediately consented to aggressive treatment. So, in order to explain that mindset we need to look at an event that happened during World War II.

Towards the end of the war, Gunther found himself in East Prussia. The war had decimated his division. Most vehicles were no longer operational. This wasn't a mechanical issue. The Germans had actually run out of gas. Gunther was left to carry his own Enigma machine, the advanced decoder of the time, while he walked with the troop line.

On April 16th, 1945 his unit was walking through an open field of tall grass. Through the rustles of the grass and the wind whistling softly in his ears, he thought he could hear a small buzzing sound. It got louder. In the distance, small tiny dots in the sky were visible. They were American planes, piloted by Soviet troops. Gunther looked around. The field was flat and there were no hills or trees to take cover under. He saw bombs falling out of the planes. With no other choice, he threw himself onto the ground.

A deafening blast followed and Gunther was thrown into the air. Before the smoke had cleared, he regained consciousness and looked to his left arm. It was pouring blood from shrapnel wounds. There was only one vehicle in the area that was intact and moving. He ran into the truck. One of his comrades drove it away to the nearest town. Gunther was transferred to a warehouse full of the wounded and propped into a tiny bed next to other troops. A medical aide came by and gave him an injection of morphine. Gunther slept and slept some more. After a while he noticed the arm had begun to change color. It smelled awful. It was developing gangrene (a condition commonly seen in severe, untreated wounds where the tissue rots from inadequate blood supply). A nurse came by and checked the arm. She gave him another injection of morphine and woke him up a little while later. He was brought into a small cellar filled with dust and told to sit down. Right across from him, a physician was operating on a wounded man who was lying on a gurney. The man had also suffered shrapnel wounds. The doctor was out of medical supplies and was poking his gloved fingers into the open flesh to pry out shrapnel.

It was Gunther's turn next. He was laid down on the gurney. The doctor looked at him and said, "I'll try to save the arm." The nurse placed a white towel on Gunther's face and he could see no more.

He woke up hours later after another man shook him from his sleep.

"We have to get going!" he said.

Gunther looked at his arm. There was a blanket over it.

"I can't go anywhere," Gunther replied hazily as he gestured to his arm.

It wasn't an option. The Soviets were about two hundred yards away. He was dragged to the last bus left in the area. As he was put into the only available seat, he heard the door slam and the bus sped away to the nearest port. Gunther was on his way to Denmark via the Baltic Sea.

Gunther can't remember much of what happened on the trip. He doesn't know if he ate at all. He slept quite a bit, and remained in his daze. With no medical gauze left, his arm was wrapped in a roll of toilet paper. During the voyage, a pastor gathered everyone's attention.

"Adolf Hitler has died in a fire in Berlin," he announced. No reactions. No sadness, no happiness. "He could have told everyone we arrived at the port, and there would have been the same reaction," Gunther remembers. "We were too exhausted to care at that point."

He arrived in Denmark, and after a train ride from Copenhagen to a small town called Nyborg, he was deposited in a school gymnasium full of the wounded soldiers who were unable to receive the proper medical treatment from across the Baltic Sea. Lying on a bed of straw, Gunther waited until a nurse made her way to him. She inspected his arm, which was still wrapped in the same toilet paper. It was full of tiny movement—maggots were crawling all over. She pulled out a pair of scissors and began to cut away at the wrapping. The scissors caught on the fabric and the nurse had to use her strength to cut through. The wrapping was mottled and had become rock hard from the mixture of aged red blood and yellow pus. The wrapping was so heavily embedded with flesh that when she cut away at the bottom she nicked an artery. Blood gurgled out and the nurse ran away to fetch a doctor. Gunther lay on the straw, watching blood gushing out of his arm. The nurse returned with a surgeon and what looked like, at least according to Gunther, two wrestlers (big guys). They pinned him down while the surgeon took out clamps. They had run out of medical supplies and this included anesthesia. Someone had to keep him still while the surgeon closed the wound. Gunther screamed as the scalpel pierced his infected flesh.

Of course, Gunther lived through all this. He even kept his arm. It's a fascinating story, but what does this have to do with cancer? Why would Gunther tell me this story when I asked him about his decision to get treatment?

Let's put the answer to that question on the back burner while we look at another war story.

Daniel was born in the small town of Warnow, Poland, an unfortunate time and place for Jewish births. By the time he was twelve, he and the rest of his family had been split into unknown regions of Poland and fed into the Nazi concentration camp system. Daniel's only fortune was not being immediately placed into a death camp.

He toiled away in a labor camp until one day a young German officer left his combat boots out in the open. The weather had been dismal, and the ground was a muddy slop staining the normally pristine Nazi uniforms. Daniel saw the dirty footwear and cleaned it up. When the officer returned, he was so impressed that he took Daniel under his wing, making him his personal assistant. Daniel's life was only moderately improved under this man's control, and though he followed him everywhere it is hard to say whether or not either of them felt an attachment.

One morning, Daniel woke up to screams. It wasn't uncommon in the camp, but this was the cry of multiple people. The "pop! pop! pop!" of machine gunfire followed and the screams stopped. Through the dirty windows of the building he slept in, Daniel saw lines of children being pushed into a ditch. He looked around at the other children inside the building. All had the same look on their faces.

They were going to die.

The officer whom he had served for so long pulled Daniel from the camp. The man showed no recognition on his face as he dragged Daniel to a ditch out by the woods. They were both silent. All around them, officers dragged young Jewish children out to the area.

When they got to the ground before the ditch, Daniel was forced to his knees. The officer leaned down and whispered into his ear. "They are forcing us to kill the boys. I'm not going to kill you, though."

He pinched Daniel's right shoulder hard. "When we've gone, run for the woods."

Daniel didn't say a word. Maybe he didn't believe him. The officer marched back several steps to a line formed by the German soldiers.

On their superior's command, they took aim.

Daniel closed his eyes.

The German commander said a word and the soldiers fired.

Daniel felt two sharp, painful jabs into his right arm and shoulder. The impact knocked him into the ditch, alongside his dead peers.

How long was he out? Who knows? All Daniel remembers is groggily climbing out of the pile of bodies and running into the woods. Dark, unknown forests were infinitely preferable to what he had lived through.

Through great fortune, Daniel was able to escape from the Nazis permanently, and eventually reunite with his family.

You see, what separates Gunther and Daniel is that one survived the war, while the other became a survivor.

We're going to cover both Gunther and Daniel's experiences with cancer in broader strokes than we have with the previous stories, because we've already gone over many of the technical details involved in their diagnosis and treatment. The real story is how they made their decisions to be treated. We'll see how their war experiences influenced their decisions on medical treatment and what it teaches us about the application of medicine to the elderly.

Gunther was diagnosed in 2009 with left-sided breast cancer. He had noticed his breast was enlarging and had become increasingly tender to the touch. It had gotten to the point where he could no longer wear even a thin shirt without being in severe pain because the fabric would put too much pressure.

He had seen this same situation before, over sixty years ago, while he was still in Germany. It was 1948 and he had gone to the doctors because the right side of his chest had swollen up, "like a woman's breast," and had become incredibly painful. Cancer was still relatively unknown—remember that chemotherapy stemmed initially from the advent of mustard gas used in World War I—and German doctors were unable to figure out what was wrong with Gunther. Their only recommendation was to cut it out, and Gunther could only thank god there was enough local anesthesia to get through it.

But that had been so long ago.

He had never seen any follow-up symptoms from either the ailment or the surgery. Yet, here he was, sixty years later in California and seeing the exact same situation play out on the opposite side. He still didn't know what he had, as his doctors in Germany had not been able to tell him.

He visited the home of a retired doctor who lived down the block. The man took a look at Gunther's chest and did a quick physical exam. "I don't think it is cancer," he told him. Gunther was told to ice it and take some painkillers.

Icing did take away some pain, and for several days the cold caused the chest swelling to decrease. It quickly ballooned again, though, and the pain was even worse this time.

It's not difficult to see why the first doctor did not think it was cancer. Cancers usually develop slowly and are usually not tender, let alone so painful that even a thin shirt will cause agony. Furthermore, breast cancer in males is not nearly as common as it is in females. (Just a side note, as we won't really be delving into male breast cancer, but BCRA, a genetic line that greatly increases the risk of breast cancer among females, is also a risk factor for males.)

Gunther finally went the extra mile, literally and figuratively, by seeing his regular primary care physician— someone who didn't live in his neighborhood. During the physical exam, the doctor pointed to the nipple on the swollen breast. "Has it been like this for a while?" he asked Gunther.

"What do you mean?" Gunther replied.

"It's turned inside-out. How long has it been like that?" the doctor pressed him.

Gunther thought about it. "I don't know. I never paid attention." The doctor pursed his lips and continued the rest of the exam. "I bet you a 100 to 1 it's cancer," he told him at the end. Gunther's whirlwind tour through the medical industry was about to begin.

He was referred to a surgeon who performed a stereotactic biopsy of his swollen breast (procedure where X-ray guidance through mammography helps pinpoint the exact location to obtain a biopsy). The biopsy confirmed that it was cancer.

He was then scheduled to have a mastectomy (lumpectomy is not done in male breast cancer, as there is minimal breast tissue and there is no breast contour to preserve). It was delayed because of a pulmonary embolism (a clot in his lungs that had most likely originated from one of his leg veins. Remember that cancer tends to thicken the blood and make a person predisposed to more clots). Finally, after a sizeable delay during which he had to take blood thinners, he was able to have a mastectomy.

The mastectomy revealed a Stage III cancer. When a large number of lymph glands are infiltrated by cancer, it is a bad prognostic sign, suggesting the chances of recurrence are extremely high. He also had the presence of ER+ and PR+ markers (estrogen and progesterone) that indicated that the cancer cells were sensitive to hormone therapy. Since his risk of recurrence was extremely high, he was started on standard chemotherapy in the form of Taxotere and Cytoxan for four cycles starting in February 2009 and completed in April 2009. He subsequently was started on hormonal therapy in the form of Tamoxifen, a pill taken once a day for five years. The role of chemotherapy in Gunther's case would be to reduce the risk of recurrence by about 20%. Tamoxifen would reduce the risk of recurrence by about 40%.

That's a lot of medical history summarized quickly, but it's enough to let us focus on the main question: should Gunther receive chemotherapy? Now, this is obviously a question that should be posed to everyone who is a candidate for it, but it becomes more complicated with Gunther's age. If he receives chemo, what is the maximum benefit he can receive, both in terms of mortality and improvement in quality of life? What will be the cost to him in terms of side effects both short term and long term? Are the side effects worth the potential benefits? If the benefits are not substantial enough to make this an obvious decision, then what are his goals in life? This refers to the question of what exactly is he living for?

Gunther has a wife but no children. Direct relatives, whether they live in the United States or abroad, will be of a similar age and also facing medical problems of their own. His wife won't be destitute, at least financially, without him. There's no birth of a grandchild or a sweet 16th birthday party that he wants to live for.

On the other hand, Gunther enjoys his life. He's retired, lives in a good community, plays golf every day, plays golf well enough so that he actually enjoys playing golf every day, and is in a general state of happiness.

Do there have to be tangible connections like children and grandchildren in order for him to be tethered to this world? According to Gunther, "Absolutely not." When he thinks now about how well he got through the treatment process, there is no doubt in his mind he made the right decision.

"Everyone has to go, and sometimes you go from an operation like I had at eighty-four. But they should treat the person until there is no more hope. I don't say that because I am eighty-five. You see, each and every person I meet says you look like, as I know you for all these years you have not changed your face, you have not lost your hair —I did, but it grew back again. They say you look the same, what are you complaining about," Gunther explains.

"That should be left up to the patient. See, I know about euthanasia. I know it is difficult to think about and talk about euthanasia because that leaves a bad taste in the mouth; I went through that after the war. However, if I were to feel...let's say I have a recurrence of the cancer in a year or two and the doctor says it was incurable. You may live only for five more months and you will be very much in pain. And we call another doctor and another one and they all say the same. Then it is left to the person who is suffering. Okay, maybe you want to live for five more months, and you will receive injections that are painful." (We'll talk about that last sentence soon.)

However, it is the suggestion that his life is not as valuable as others simply because of age that agitates Gunther. It's the reason he loves to tell the story of how he survived the bombings by the Soviets.

"I have gone through more than one instance in my life which was threatened," he begins. "Look at it this way, as a young person you can be sent to war and your life is worth nothing if you get killed. So how much more worth is an older man's life than a younger man's life? You cannot set an amount on it. If you do, that is a business condition. And I feel that should be left alone."

The point is, as Gunther puts it- how much "value" was there in his life as a twenty-year-old? Consider the hypothetical situation where there are two patients who come into a cancer clinic at the same time with the exact same cancer, only one is twenty years old and the other is eighty-five. And there is only enough of the chemotherapy drug to treat one of them. Who is the more deserving of the two? The traditional reasoning, if one is forced to make a decision, is the younger person has more years ahead of them, and therefore the "value" of their life is greater. But as Gunther saw it, during his time in the war, he had no expectation to live a long life. His chance of dying, per year, as a twenty-year-old, was just as great, if not greater, as his chance of dying now in his ripened age.

So do soldiers—or, say, a drug officer on the southern borders of the United States, or any other people placed in hazardous conditions also fall in the same category as the elderly when it comes to determining treatment? Okay, so you can always quit your job. The military won't send out cancer-ridden troops to fight, whereas the elderly can't reverse their age.

Let's assess "value" in another way then. When Ted Kennedy, the late Massachusetts senator, was diagnosed with an incurable brain tumor, he was able to assemble a world-class team of specialists to confer on treatment options within a week.

Despite his age, and the fact that the disease was incurable, he received the necessary treatment to prolong his life. So, if you're a physician, and a United States senator comes into your office dying from a terminal cancer, you're not going to counsel a course of action that includes no pharmaceutical help. What if the senator is ninety years old? Does age no longer matter with a VIP? How exactly are we determining value?

What about a young male growing up in a gang-infested area of a city like Detroit or Chicago? By some estimates, the average life expectancy of a gang member is a little over twenty years old. That's a survival rate that corresponds well to the rates of attrition for most elderly. While a solider or officer can quit their job, that immediate opportunity is not afforded to the destitute (they may or may not climb out of poverty, but that ascension will not happen immediately). So would anyone suggest an eighteen-year-old male gang member, who lives on the west side of Chicago, not be offered treatment for a leukemia simply because his chance of death is so great within the next few years? Is present and future worth as a citizen an indication to not be treated?

On the other hand, can't there be at least some argument to be made for not being treated?

"I've heard the other sides," Gunther says. He gives the story of a morning when he joined a friend for a game of golf. Gunther was more of an acquaintance than a close friend, and hadn't yet revealed his diagnosis. When he did, the conversation immediately turned to whether or not he should go through with the treatment.

"What would you do?" Gunther asked him as they set their clubs down by the tee off.

The friend, over ninety years old at that point, carefully set his ball on the tee. It was a warm, beautiful day in Northern California and the two of them were enjoying everything they had despite the nature of the conversation. "Gunther, I would not have gone through this chemo. But my wife passed away, so whom do I live for? You still have a wife, so you may have a different opinion than I do."

"So I have heard other sides," Gunther explains.

What would medical professionals think about encouraging someone of his age not to receive full treatment? His oncologist bristled at the idea of someone other than the patient making the decision.

"As far as I am concerned, any plans that put restrictions on the amount of care that can be provided by insurance companies or the federal government is absurd. These decisions are being made by people who are young and healthy. These decisions are made based on arrogance of power and hubris. Just because you are in a position of power in the healthcare field, that does not mean you have a right to decide who gets what care and who does not. These decisions need to be made by the patient after being well informed of all the different options. The HMOs and managed care organizations at present restrict care, but that choice is made by the patient to join an HMO based on their financial constraints. I feel that is fine. But for the federal government to mandate that patients go into managed care is absurd. If they or their loved ones had a serious illness, the song they sing would be completely different."

"Listen, I worked in England for a couple of years. They have a wonderful healthcare system, but there are restrictions and restraints. But, they do not apply to the people in power. When I was there, if you had a heart attack and were one day above the age of sixty-five years, you would be admitted to a regular medical floor without any heart monitors. If you were one day below the age of sixty-five years, you would be admitted to a monitored/intensive care unit. How silly and ridiculous. But that's how it was. I do not know if the same situation still exists. I cannot imagine a politician or somebody powerful being admitted after a heart attack to a non-intensive care floor. These are obviously complex issues. There are no completely right answers, but there are a number of wrong answers. All I say is that all the politicians, their families, and their children should have the same restrictions that they promote," the oncologist said.

Gunther chose chemotherapy and did well. Let's take a look at Daniel's story before we discuss the after effects of both men's choices. One thing I would like to make clear is that in reviewing the account from Daniel and his relatives, and the actual written record constituting his medical charts—there were differences. This is not to suggest that any side is lying, but perception can severely distort each person's account. Why Daniel made an initial choice not to be treated is not as important as the fact that he made it.

Daniel, at the age of seventy-seven, was already a survivor of cancer. He had been diagnosed with colon cancer in 2001 and the experience with the medical industry had been less than satisfactory. To those who knew him well, this was not a surprise.

His experiences in World War II had transformed him into a permanent nihilist.

It helped explain why he could never trust authority. Daniel had resolved to be as fully independent as possible. An engineer, he quickly ascended the ranks in his company and became manager to over one hundred people. He was used to calling the shots. His philosophy on life would complicate the relationship between him and his physicians. Daniel would not be happy letting the outcome of his life be determined by a small group of people. He would not want to live life unless it was a good quality one. This attitude would limit his treatment options, especially in the face of an ailment like cancer. He was also part of an HMO that will go unnamed in this story. Whether or not you feel the HMO is a blessing or curse to medical industry, no one denies there are limitations to the treatment plans available. That is to say, for people who truly want every option available and a full scope of independence when it comes to their health, there are better options than most HMOs.

"He has a persecution complex—he doesn't want to be beholden to anybody. All these things were done to him against his will. Almost a post-traumatic stress disorder. Very frightened of situations where someone else is in control, when he has to be dependent on other people he becomes paranoid. They think you're hurting them, that you're tricking them," his daughter explains. You see, Daniel's attitude doesn't apply only to strangers, but even friends and family, some of whom (his daughter and son-in-law) work in the medical industry.

It would play out in a major way when, at the age of seventy-seven, he was diagnosed with a squamous cell carcinoma at the base of the tongue.

Eight years after his bout of colon cancer, he called his daughter to ask about a strange symptom. His throat had been sore for the past six months. He also had bad breath that wouldn't go away no matter how much he brushed, chewed gum, or mouthwashed. At first, his daughter chalked it up to a dental condition. Daniel, despite being well off, had no dental insurance and had not seen a dentist in over fifteen years. Halitosis made sense. "I dragged him to the dentist, like a child," she laughs. His teeth were bronzed. "We wanted to see if his teeth were only stained or discolored or if they were rotten."

The dentist was suspicious about the examination, and there was certainly nothing in the exam that truly explained his symptoms. He was referred for some more diagnostics and in April he was told he had cancer in the base of the tongue.

He called up his daughter to tell her the news.

"Base of the tongue?" she asked. "Can you swallow?

"It's getting difficult," he replied. He talked a little bit more about the problems he was having and then he said something that sent chills up his daughter's spine. He had made a decision. He wasn't going to receive treatment for the cancer. "I don't think it can be treated. It's going to kill me. I think I'm going to die from this."

"Daddy, you don't have to die from this," his daughter replied, utterly perplexed by his statement "And even if you die, there's better ways to go—it's better to starve to death than to die from a choking, bleeding death, asphyxiation."

"I don't want to be disabled like your mother. I've been told that they can't help me, that nothing can be done," he answered in a tone that suggested this was a final decision.

"Why are you saying this? It's just not true." She begged him to let her consult specialists on his condition.

Now, there is nothing on the paper record, the documentation of his initial office visits with the oncologists at his HMO, to suggest they flatly denied any chance for survival. But what is said and how things are said are two very different matters. Is it quite possible Daniel misunderstood their recommendations. It is quite possible his physicians looked at his overall condition including his age and said, "Maybe it's better to not undergo any treatment." In most HMOs, the less you do, the more money you make. So the bias is to do less. It is quite possible they explored every option, but their tone was most favorable to a no treatment path. It is possible he received advice from other sources, including other close family and friends that warped his perception of the doctor's advice. Again, the truth lies somewhere in between all accounts. We'll look at it from the view of Daniel and his family, mostly because it allows us to explore a contrast to Gunther's story.

Daniel, at the time of his diagnosis, had three treatment options. He could have had open head and neck surgery in an effort to dissect out the cancer. Given the sensitive nature of the afflicted area, this would be a limited surgery and likely require follow-up either by chemotherapy, radiation, or both. This was an option, if you recall Peter's story that had been rejected in a much younger, healthier man who had cancer around the same region.

A second option would be to get eight weeks of radiation.

Finally he could have a combination approach of chemotherapy and eight weeks of radiation. This would be the option recommended to most people—this would have the highest chance of curing the disease, but would cause many side effects.

So, just as we explored the context of Gunther's condition, let us do the same thing with Daniel. Should he be treated? What would a round of chemotherapy and radiation do for him both in terms of quality of life and mortality? What is he living for? Furthermore, what would prompt Daniel to not receive any treatment?

If you look at his social situation, Daniel provides an interesting contrast to Gunther. He actually has children (and grandchildren), along with other family in the country. He was married, and had divorced his children's mother some time before she developed Alzheimer's. Like Gunther, he was comfortable financially. Both were in reasonable states of health and had good prognosis with the administration of treatment. What could prompt one to jump for treatment and the other to refuse it? At that point you look at either philosophy in life or the manner in which all this information is conveyed to them.

Daniel needed more than just assurance of cure. First, he wanted brevity of treatment. Long therapy and follow-up represented loss of authority to him. His life would constantly be under the control of a medical provider and he wanted no part of that.

He wanted a good quality of life after the treatment. His standards in this matter were high. Years before, when he had developed a colon cancer, he had almost refused operations to remove the tumor until his surgeons assured him he would not have to live with an ostomy bag (these are prosthetic collection devices attached to a colon to collect stool, only they reside on the outside of the body. While they certainly lower quality of life, most people will choose to live with them rather than die). He had seen his ex-wife debilitated from Alzheimer's and told his daughter he would not be living like that. Debilitation through surgery, chemo, or radiation would not be acceptable.

Finally, he wanted assurances and not just optimistic predictions. This was perhaps the area that frustrated his daughter the most. As with all other people we've covered, Daniel wasn't getting information only from his physicians, but any other person who knew of his condition. Anecdotes, harmless on their own, would only serve to confuse more. And assuring medical treatment sans complication is deception. If you remember Vanessa's story, there is no free lunch in medicine.

Now, aside from preserving life, what else is the benefit of treatment? At least initially the quality of life deteriorates, with the side effects of radiation therapy and chemotherapy. This includes burning and pain in the mouth and neck—the pain can be quite severe, causing difficulty in eating; most patients end up requiring a feeding tube inserted through the wall of the abdomen for feeding, but after the initial side effects of treatment gradually taper off the quality of life improves in a major fashion. The pain is less, eating is easier although dry mouth persists.

A quick check with specialists confirmed the suspicions of Daniel's daughter and son-in-law: the disease absolutely was treatable in a way that satisfied all his demands. They just couldn't understand what was prompting him to refuse it.

Daniel stubbornly refused to discuss the matter.

Then in April, his daughter received the following email:

"Hi Everyone,

First of all we want to thank all of you who have called and emailed me with your caring and love, and tell you how much we appreciate it and that we return love to you. Your calls and emails mean so much to us.

Unfortunately, we have bad news to report. The cancer in (Daniel)'s body has spread. The doctors have given him two to six months to live. Therefore he has chosen not to have chemotherapy or radiation, but to die with dignity.

First we are going north to be with our children. Then we are going to Costa Rica for a week. We shall return home late on May 15....

We wish the news could be better.

-(Daniel) and (His wife)"

This was a goodbye letter.

Shortly after she saw the email, her dad called her to let her know he would be making the six-hour drive to come see her in North California.

This was going to be the goodbye visit.

His daughter was ready. It was clear Daniel had considered her and her husband to be biased sources. In his mind, they were giving medical opinions influenced by their heavy desire to see him live. What they needed was for him to actually hear out other medical professionals that had no connection to him.

His daughter organized a "coincidental" meeting with one of their friends who happened to be an oncologist.

Daniel was not too keen on treatment. "What's the point? You can't live forever and I don't need my life to be prolonged."

His wife was also not too keen on treatment.

"He's too old for treatment," she would tell people.

But the point of treatment was not just to cure the disease, but also to improve quality of life and prevent painful complications. The oncologist expanded on this for Daniel.

"The issue to me really is quality of life. Just because you are elderly and wish to die does not mean you are suddenly going to die if you do not take any treatment. The process of dying takes time, and that does not mean that your quality of life is going to be better. Often without treatment the disease will progress and burrow and invade into the surrounding structures, leading to significant pain and discomfort. Radiation treatment can help prevent such complications, so the goal of treatment would not just be to prolong life, but to maintain a reasonable quality of life, at the expense of the side effects of treatment which may be more tolerable than the complications of progression of disease."

It was the first time Daniel had heard about the diminished morbidity, not just mortality, that would ensue without treatment.

The oncologist went into more detail by explaining, "The cancer slowly continues to grow, leading to pain, bleeding, bad breath, difficulty in swallowing. A person can slowly bleed to death, can gradually starve to death, the tumor can erode through the base of the skull leading to intractable pain and discomfort. So if you do not take treatment, it does not mean you can turn off a switch and die. It is a slow, lingering, painful death, with the potential for many different complications. With treatment there is a high chance of shrinking the disease for a certain length of time, and about a 30% chance of getting rid of the disease completely."

But won't this happen anyway if the treatments don't work or in cases where the cancer is incurable?

"Not necessarily," the oncologist explains. "Without the treatment, the chances of those painful symptoms are 100%. Let's pretend that it is incurable, though. With treatment, you have a chance of controlling the local symptoms from the cancer amassing in one particular area, while it stills spreads systemically throughout the body. That systemic spread will be what eventually kills the person. You're not guaranteed to control the local, very painful symptoms—but the chances are better than 0% as compared to not taking any treatment."

Daniel's daughter had subsequently arranged for him to have a second opinion by a radiation oncologist who was an expert on this type of cancer and was not part of the HMO. He also stated and explained to the patient that the disease was potentially treatable and curable, albeit with certain short-term and perhaps some long-term side effects. Daniel now suddenly had opinions from three people (including his son-in-law) who all stated this disease was treatable and curable. His HMO had offered the treatment but had not been pushy about it. Now he was feeling the heat to change his mind.

He finally agreed to the treatment. He chose chemotherapy and radiation therapy.

He went through the treatment quite well except for radiation burns to his neck and his mouth. The radiation burns were quite painful, but they were temporary. These gradually improved and he subsequently returned to his usual normal active life, except for changes in his taste and dry mouth. He also has to visit his dentist every two months. His physicians told him he would lose all of his teeth. He did not lose any. Incredibly, almost every one of Daniel's desires had been fulfilled.

A few months after completing his treatment, he was feeling quite well and decided to drive all the way from southern California to his daughter's house in northern California. He had been off recently and he couldn't pinpoint a reason. He felt like he couldn't move as well as usual and he certainly didn't feel like his normal sharp self.

On the street before his daughter's house, there was a checkpoint that provided security for the neighborhood. Daniel had gone through it numerous times. Some of the guards recognized him now. As he slowed his car while hooking left, Daniel pulled into the leftmost lane to talk to the guard. Only he never stopped his vehicle. He drove straight through the gate, cracking the windshield and breaking the barrier. The curbside finally broke the momentum of his car.

Daniel had suffered a stroke that confused and debilitated him. His anti-cholesterol medications and aspirin had been discontinued at the time of treatment and had not been restarted at its completion. Without these medications, he was more susceptible to ischemic (lack of blood flow to an area due to either a clot or narrowing of the blood vessels) incidents and had sustained a stroke.

More than the debilitation from the stroke, Daniel was angry because he felt he was misled. His worst nightmare was a crippling mental or physical injury. It was what he strived to avoid most, and the reason he had been okay with death from the cancer. Yet, here he was, supposedly "cured" and worse off than he had been with a terminal illness. Imagine how he felt in those initial moments of diagnosis and debilitation. It would have been understandable to be angry at all those who promised him it would work out, from his son-in-law to the oncologists.

Since then, Daniel has recovered, but not completely. He still gets intermittently confused and is unable to drive at present. He has had mild memory loss and some cognitive issues. His cancer remains in remission.

It's difficult for me to really agree with how he feels. This could have happened without the treatment. I also think this is a far better scenario than what would have occurred without the treatment, but then again it's up for him to decide that. What is clear, though, is that his cancer was curable.

Now, these are all thoughts from Gunther and Daniel. What would an oncologist, like the family friend who spoke to Daniel, someone who has seen numerous people like these two in his practice, think about the decision to receive chemotherapy?

He answered by explaining his approach to patients. "I start off the way I would with any patient, giving all the possible options. By this time I have an idea of the patient's physiological age as compared to the chronological age. I lay out the side effects of treatment and the potential benefits. I then simply ask the patient what they would like to do. Most patients opt for the standard treatment, whatever their age. In my opinion that's the way it should be. It is very difficult to put myself in the boots of somebody who is elderly. Everybody has different experiences in life. My job is to give them information and knowledge I have because of my education and experience, so they can make informed decisions. I do help guide the decision-making process, but I try not to make decisions for them. I give them options."

He continued, "Listen, nobody wants to die unless they are really miserable. Our Darwinian brain is wired to fight for survival. That is how we survive…maybe I want to live for one more year to see my grandson born, or I want to live one more year to see my daughter get married, or maybe I want to live because I like living as my quality of life is reasonable to me."

He recalled one patient whose story stuck with him. "There was another lady who was eighty-nine years old who had an aggressive breast cancer. She walked into the office, and told me specifically to treat her like a 65-year-old. She had never been ill before. Her quality of life was very good; she loved spending time with her grandchildren, and told me she was not ready to die yet. She went through chemotherapy and Herceptin. I wanted to give her chemo that was not as aggressive, but she asked for the full cycle, and she actually did better than most women younger than her. I remember her distinctly as she and I had the same birthday. She would always send me a card on my birthday and always called to chat with me. She unfortunately died three years later of a different cancer unrelated to the breast cancer—pancreatic cancer. But she was always grateful for the extra three years she had with her children and grandchildren. I learnt a lot from that experience, and often quote her to my older patients."

What do we make of these opinions? Of Gunther and Daniel's experiences? Or for that matter, any of the other patients we have covered?

First off, I understand there is no imminent push toward concepts such as death panels. Hopefully we will never move in that direction. But the way we treat our elderly and approach their issues is representative of this country's medical system. There are other ways to create casualties in healthcare besides denial of treatment. Our priorities by and large determine the best outcomes. We see a problem, and focus our energy, brains, and money to fix it to the best of our abilities. Sometimes it works well, like with the war on breast cancer...sometimes spectacularly, like the eradication of smallpox. But when we shift our resources, it is only inevitable that other illnesses get neglected.

The geriatric population is growing and will continue to demand more attention and time. Whether or not it is in our interest to focus on them, whether it is moral to do that or not to do that, I can't tell. The Macmillan Cancer Support Organization of Great Britain came out with a report in 2013 that demonstrated numerous elderly patients were not being given sufficient care when it came to cancers. While the mortality rate of malignancy had dropped in almost every age group over the past several decades, it had actually increased among the elderly. The authors of the report were concerned about the attitude of physicians to look at the numerical age of the patient, instead of their overall fitness and life goals, to determine they shouldn't receive full treatment.

It's not as if physicians in England got together in a conference to arrange this attitude. It's probably not even a conscious effort on the individual level. But somewhere in the system is a facet that is worsening care for the elderly. Maybe it's a necessity. England's medical system on the whole does a great job at providing care for the entire country. Every system has flaws, and perhaps this is an acceptable one.

But I know after meeting with Gunther and Daniel that as a young man, not in their well-worn shoes, it would take extreme hubris to decide the right choices for them.

Cancer is difficult to deal with, and not just because it is a terminal disease. That fact is obviously a big component, but the other significant piece of the puzzle is cancer forces everyone to make difficult decisions. Within the scope of the patient, each person's decisions are of a different nature.

For example, the physician's decisions are medical. They have to be made scientifically and logically. The patient has to be informed of all the options and the rationale behind the options. The pros and cons of different plans need to be discussed. The issue with these decisions is the physician automatically processes the information into a conclusion. It is easy for them to do this. They have years of experience with the cognitive decision-making process. For the patient, though, this is a completely new and frightening experience. One of the most common statements uttered to the oncologist is: "This is all very new to me and I don't understand."

Then the family members and their perspective come in to play. They mean well, but give advice based on anecdotes, in fear, rather than logic and science. Intuition comes in. It can be wrong just as often as it can be right. More importantly, they have the ear of the patient. Why wouldn't you trust your friends and family? After all, they just want to see you do well.

Of course, the medical system in general has decisions to make. As in Daniel's case, HMOs provide a network at reduced costs, but restrict the options. Hospitals can lean on physicians to be more accepting of some treatments over others.

Most importantly, the patients themselves have decisions to make—decisions that stem from a value system that up until the diagnosis may not have been fully clear. The prognosis or treatability of the cancer type doesn't matter because once you have cancer, *any cancer*, your previous life is irretrievable. That threat of cancer is there permanently and now you have to make the decision of how to live life in that new universe. In these stories, each person leaves their stamp on the illness by the way they want to go through life.

Mike wanted to live long enough to see events—from Christmas to the birth of a grandson. Marty had to honor the promise to his father to be strong. Vanessa needed peace of mind. Peter never wanted to be a guinea pig for other physicians. Jenny didn't want cancer to force her into marriage or subservience to Western medicine. Whether it is their optimism, their desire for control, their distrust of authority, each of them views the disease and the healthcare industry through their unique personal prism. Their struggles come either from obstacles preventing them from maintaining that frame, or doubts about that frame's benefit to their life.

Balancing and processing all of these cognitive inputs is not exactly easy for most people. This book is a portrayal of choices made and their consequences. There is often information overload. Sorting them out takes time and support. One thing is certain— decisions should be made by individuals and not by faceless management through the healthcare industry and the government. The decision-makers have to be the ones with their feet near the fire.

What may be rational to us may not be rational to the patient.

When we recommend decisions to others, due to age or other factors, we've done so through our own way of looking at life. For most of us, that includes a vision originating from a universe not altered by malignancy. It is ignorant to tell people that they shouldn't live life in the way they want to. Cancer has already robbed of them vitality; now we deprive them of autonomy.

Imagine what it feels like to spend your whole life fighting, fighting, fighting; whether it is in the service of others or happiness for yourself. And then, in the most desperate moments of your life, near the end, you are kicked to the curb…not because others wouldn't fight the cancer, but because they can't imagine you fighting it. They can't see the point. The point isn't for them to see. It's for the patient's vision only.

One last thing.

Of the original nine patients I interviewed, only four are still alive.

Two of them include Gunther and Daniel. Their ages at present are eighty-eight and eighty-two, respectively.

Of course, it's just anecdotal. I caught some patients at times when the cancer had just broken through, and some who were beyond fortunate in the way they responded to treatment. But I told you in the beginning I wasn't big on statistics. And every year that Gunther and Daniel keep chugging along is another reason why.

CPSIA information can be obtained
at www.ICGtesting.com
Printed in the USA
BVHW040347210221
600563BV00005B/18

9 781478 754831